OSCEs for Medical Students, Volume 1
Second Edition

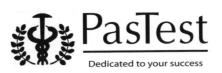

PasTest

Dedicated to your success

OSCEs for Medical Students, Volume 1
Second Edition

Adam Feather

John S P Lumley

Ramanathan Visvanathan

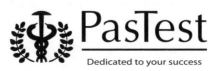

PasTest

Dedicated to your success

© 2004 PASTEST Ltd
Egerton Court
Parkgate Estate
Knutsford
Cheshire
WA16 8DX

Telephone: 01565 752000

First published 2004, reprinted 2006, 2007, 2008

ISBN: 1 904627 09 9
ISBN: 978 1 904627 09 8

A catalogue record for this book is available from the British Library.

The information contained within this book was obtained by the authors from reliable sources. However, while every effort has been made to ensure its accuracy, no responsibility for loss, damage or injury occasioned to any person acting or refraining from action as a result of information contained herein can be accepted by the publishers or authors.

PasTest Revision Books and Intensive Courses
PasTest has been established in the field of postgraduate medical education since 1972, providing revision books and intensive study courses for doctors preparing for their professional examinations.

Books and courses are available for the following specialties:
MRCGP, MRCP Parts 1 and 2, MRCPCH Parts 1 and 2, MRCPsych, MRCS, MRCOG Parts 1 and 2, DRCOG, FRCA, PLAB Parts 1 and 2.

For further details contact:
PasTest, Knutsford, Cheshire WA16 7BR
Tel: 01565 752000   Fax: 01565 650264
www.pastest.co.uk   enquiries@pastest.co.uk

Text prepared by Carnegie Book Production, Lancaster
Printed and bound by Cambridge University Press, Cambridge, UK

Contents

OSCE Stations

Answers with Explanations and Comments

Contributors

Adam Feather MB MRCP
Senior Lecturer in Medical Education
St Bartholomew's and The Royal London Hospital Medical School
Consultant Physician
Newham Healthcare Trust
London

John S P Lumley MS FRCS
Professor of Vascular Surgery
University of London
Honorary Consultant Surgeon
Great Ormond Street Children's Hospital
Medical College and Hospital of St Bartholomew, London
Member of Council, Royal College of Surgeons of England
Past World President, International College of Surgeons

Ramanathan Visvanathan BM BCh FRCS ILTM
Consultant Surgeon
Bronglais General Hospital
Aberystwyth
SY23 1ER
And Breast Test Wales, Swansea
Honorary Lecturer, University of Wales College of Medicine
Surgical Tutor, Royal College of Surgeons of England

Angela Hall BSc Postgrad DipSoc
Senior Lecturer in Clinical Communications
Department of Medical Health Care Education
St George's Hospital Medical School
Cranmer Terrace
Tooting
London
SW17 0RE

Acknowledgements

These volumes would not have reached their present high standards without the excellent contribution made by Angela Hall, Senior Lecturer in Communication Skills at St George's Hospital Medical School. Her expert advice on the process elements of all the communication skills stations have improved the quality and have helped to produce stations which truly reflect those used at the majority of UK medical schools at final MBBS. Whilst the style of OSCE checklists will no doubt evolve over the next few years the elements she has included will not. We are very grateful to her for her expert contribution.

Preface

Followers of recent literature on the assessment of undergraduate medical training could be excused for thinking that traditional methods were incomplete, if not arbitrary, and that potentially harmful doctors were being let loose on an unsuspecting public. This opinion is based on the immeasurable nature of 'gut feeling' in the marking of an essay and assessing clinical competence. The application of objective measurement in qualifying examinations does add credibility to their outcome.

Every examination must be fair and favour the well-prepared, ie valid and reliable. We have discussed the relative merits of essays, SAQs and MCQs elsewhere, this book, (and its companion volumes), is directed at the use of OSCEs in medicine. It provides a means of assessing practical procedures and communication skills, as well as knowledge and attitudes in most aspects of training.

The book is aimed at students preparing for their exit examination and will provide experience in this now widely-used examination technique. The book will also help those setting OSCE questions, providing a template onto which they can develop their own themes. OSCEs can assess history, examination, investigation and treatment of disease, together with practical techniques. OSCE stations can also obtain information on attitudes, interpersonal skills and ethical opinions. Some of these stations require the use of standard patients, manikin and videos. Although these media are not all reproduceable in a text book, advice is given on the way to deal with the likely questions, techniques and style of stations that may be encountered. It indicates what the examiner is looking for and how marks are being allocated for the approach to a patient and empathy with their problem. A correct diagnosis is not necessarily the key to obtaining a satisfactory mark: always remember to read the instructions very carefully.

The book follows a systems approach and each chapter includes questions from each type of OSCE station. Space is left for the student to respond to each question. Answers and additional advice are given in a separate section, allowing the students to assess their performance and identify areas needing further attention. In keeping with other books in the series, a revision checklist is given, and mock examinations are laid out: these latter can be undertaken within a prescribed time schedule and used for self-assessment.

Preface to the Second Edition

A chapter of paediatric stations and an extended chapter in obstetrics and gynaecology have been added in these new editions, increasing the series to three volumes. At the request of students, checklists have been included at the beginning of each chapter and there have been minor stylistic changes.

The marking system in most undergraduate examinations is item-based, although many schools are moving towards the standard postgraduate domain-based assessment, such as of generic skills and examining a region of the body; the text reflects these changing practices.

An interesting and desirable development has been the move back towards structured short cases, with emphasis on diagnostic skills, rather than process. The text also reflects these changes, as seen from the additional examiner's questions in many stations.

Units have not been included in the questions but tables of normal values are included at the beginning of each volume.

Introduction

Traditional methods of assessing knowledge and clinical skills have been based on the essay and MCQ, for written tests, and the long cases, short cases and the viva for practical aspects. These forms of assessment have been extensively challenged as to their ability to test and rank students. The essay has come under the greatest criticism but the long and short cases have also been questioned as to their objectivity and reliability. Marking a viva can be very subjective and it provides a very patchy assessment of the curriculum.

Objective structured clinical examinations (OSCEs) have been designed to provide a broader coverage of knowledge and skills in a quantifiable, valid and reliable form. They aim to assess interpretive skills, as well as factual recall; they include task-orientated items and they can examine a candidate's powers of decision making and their behavioural attitude in simulated professional practice. The overall effect is to provide a more valid assessment of candidates for their subsequent clinical practice.

The OSCE comprises a number of stations, through which a group of students rotate. The number of students in the examination usually matches the number of stations, so that by the end of the examination, each student has visited every station. There may be more stations than candidates without disturbing the organisation of the examination. Usually the time allowed for each station is the same throughout but it can be increased by inserting rest or preparatory stations before a longer question. Rest stations may also be used to provide natural breaks and to increase the number of candidates being examined at any one time.

The time at a station is usually at least three minutes, five minutes being common; 24 stations are available for a two hour examination. For an examination to be statistically reliable there must be a minimum of 17–20 stations. Formative assessments may use a few selected stations (eg 5–10). The design of OSCE questions is usually only limited by the ingenuity of the examiners. However, questions should examine a specific part of the curriculum, rather than just an ability to respond to the style of the examination. Students should be exposed to all proposed designs of question format before the final examination.

Each station of an OSCE should assess a discrete skill. This may be a basic test of practical ability or knowledge, or involve a higher level of thinking. It is wise to have a range of difficulty to help discriminate within a group. A number of questions are included to assess core knowledge: all students are expected to pass these stations. The clinical skills of diagnosis and treatment can be divided up into:

- taking a history
- performing an examination
- requesting appropriate investigations
- making the diagnosis
- assessing the severity of the disease
- prescribing treatment.

The latter should incorporate all aspects of care, including medicine, surgery, nursing and other medical and paramedical disciplines.

The history may be taken from a standardised patient (SP), or presented as a written scenario or a video. SPs may be simulated or actual patients. In the former, a well individual is trained to simulate a patient's illness in a standard way, portraying a patient's problems. Some training is usually required for actual patients, to ensure that the main points are brought out on request and that a history can be covered fully within the time allowed for that station. Simulated patients are usually actors, although sometimes students may act as SPs. In so doing students learn the evaluation process by direct observation and listening to presentations. These stations are usually manned by an examiner who is watching and listening, not only to the style of questioning, but also to student/patient interrelationships, their conversational skills, interpersonal skills, behaviour, attitude and psychomotor assessment. SPs are often asked to give their marks on the student encounter. Written scenarios can form the basis of subsequent questions, along the line of structured answer questions. They can test factual knowledge, understanding and cognitive skills but assess clinical competencies to a variable extent. Well-trained actors can become skilled historians and very persuasive patients, such as when replicating a psychiatric disturbance, although the latter are often more effectively covered with video sequences.

Examination of a patient in a manned station is a very valuable form of assessment. However, it also presents a great problem to the examiner, since very few conditions can be repeatedly examined for two hours at a time, and the number of conditions that can be easily replicated is limited, particularly if there are a number of groups of students being examined simultaneously or consecutively. Fit models can be used for the demonstration of a normal examination and normal anatomy or, alternatively, manikins can be available to assess specific examination techniques such as rectal and vaginal assessment.

A text book has difficulty in reproducing a history and examination, in view of their practical nature and the requirement of simulated patients, videos and models. This book does, however, consider the likely SPs, historical scenarios and types of models and manikins, and the examination techniques that are encountered in OSCEs. Investigations and their interpretation can easily be presented in OSCE form, and candidates can expect charts, and lists of haematological and biochemical results, together with all forms of radiological investigations, with a request to interpret data and radiological abnormalities.

OSCE stations are suitable for most aspects of treatment and prognosis. It is essential to remember that treatment of a 'medical' illness should not be limited to drugs or that of a 'surgical' illness to surgery alone. They should include all forms of available and desirable intervention. This avoids the 'pigeon-holing' of disease entities into conventional specialities which is deprecated in current clinical teaching. Counselling skills and the assessment of ethical factors in clinical practice are readily tested in an OSCE setting as SPs can provide both the background and the patient's attitude to an illness. The practical application of clinical skills and procedures are also readily assessed, usually with the aid of a manikin which allows such procedures as venous catheterization, cardiopulmonary resuscitation, securing and maintaining an air-way, wound debridement and suturing.

Desirable Features of OSCEs

OSCEs bring a new dimension to the assessment of medical training. Of particular value is their ability to examine practical and other skills in a unified, measurable and reproducible fashion. This is in keeping with current trends towards performance based assessment throughout health care. OSCEs provide for an effective use of the examination time, examiners' time and commitment. They are effective in assessing knowledge and practical skills and ensure that each student is presented with the same material, thus providing a uniform evaluation with consistent marking of all those involved.

The validity of the response to each question is primarily related to the student's ability: in well constructed questions, very little variation is dependent on the examiner's responses in manned stations. The reliability of OSCEs in differentiating good from bad students and the inter-rater reliability of examiners is good, and becomes increasingly certain as the number of stations devoted to each component part is increased. Both construct and content validity have been well established.

Well constructed questions are durable and can stand up to repeated use without weakening their value. Like many forms of assessment, effective questions represent the core curriculum material, and once a suitable bank size has been achieved, security of the questions is unnecessary as knowledge of the answers represents a passable understanding of the curriculum. Experiments on presenting a single station at a time to groups of students have not reduced their value in differentiating clinical performance. Assessment can be by the students themselves or by peer review. This modification substantially reduces the necessary space and organisation for an OSCE.

OSCEs can be a useful teaching modality. With the reduced stay of patients in hospitals and increased community-based education, medical schools often have to extend their teaching practice onto a number of sites. All these factors increase the need for uniformity of teaching methods as well as assessment. This can be effectively achieved with the use of OSCEs, and the reduced number of available patients can be addressed by the use of standard patients with good effect. One well-proven example of the use of simulated patients has been in the training and assessment of trauma, linked to the Advanced Trauma Life Support and related programmes. The use of students as SPs has proved an important and enjoyable learning experience, as well as, in some cases, providing financial rewards.

- Construct validity is the ability of the OSCE to differentiate students' ability, or to follow a student's progress before and after a course of instruction.
- Content (criterion-based) validity assesses the value of the station in reaching its specified objective. In all these measures OSCEs have proved effective in student assessment and are accepted by staff and students as a fair and desirable form of assessment.

Assessment is a powerful learning tool and should be used as part of the teaching and learning processes but it must be accompanied by adequate feedback in order to benefit individual students. This process should also be used in auditing teaching methods and to stimulate any necessary changes. It is feasible to set up OSCEs in any medical school, provided appropriate staff time is allowed for their introduction. Some schools involve students in the design and development of OSCEs and it can increase their awareness of this form of assessment. The formulation of OSCEs should be closely linked with curriculum development and keyed into the curriculum objectives.

When using OSCEs to evaluate teaching methods, two types of error should be considered.

- Type I errors are those of fact, implying a deficiency of teaching and/or learning, reflecting omissions and ineffective or absent experience.
- Type II errors are defects of understanding, where a student fails to recognise or interpret a clinical situation. This reflects poor concept attainment and an inability to discriminate.

Locating these errors points to the direction that future teaching should follow.

Disadvantages of OSCEs

As discussed in the previous section, the value of OSCEs in training and assessment has been demonstrated in many fields and many such assessment packages are available. However, medical schools should not become involved in this form of assessment without allowing adequate staff time for their development and OSCEs should not become the only form of assessment.

The preparation of OSCEs requires a good deal of thought and time. The whole staff should be aware of, and preferably involved in, their development and students should have experience prior to any examination so that they can be comfortable with this form of assessment. An OSCE requires a great deal of organisation in collecting material, appropriate patients, laying out stations and making sure staff are available for manned areas. Setting up the examination can be costly on administration and on medical staff and patients, and includes the hidden costs of Faculty time in the development of the exercise.

Analysis of the data and ensuring the validity of the examination requires painstaking activity. The weighting of key questions on essential knowledge has to be resolved before any feedback to staff or students. Standard setting should be based on expected knowledge and the skills required and this relies as much on that much-criticized 'gut feeling' as it does on statistical formulae. Standardised patients, both actual and simulated have to be found and trained and an adequate pool must be available to cover expected needs. When introducing OSCEs, a school has to decide whether it is as an additional assessment or whether it should replace a previous part of the examination. If the latter, it is essential that other important areas are not diluted in the process. OSCEs are not ideal in assessing interpersonal skills: video clips or trained patients can be rather artificial in this respect. For patient examination, OSCEs do not provide a comprehensive evaluation of all aspects of a learning and educational programme and therefore should be part of a multi-component assessment in the final examination, forming a useful means of determining practical skills over a wide area.

In spite of their potential limitations, OSCEs do provide a valuable addition to the clinical exit examination and students and staff should become well acquainted with their format and appreciate their discriminatory properties.

How to Use this Book

This book contains a series of OSCE questions. The chapters are arranged by organ system, and every chapter follows the same organisation of questions, i.e. history, examination, investigation, treatment, practical techniques and other issues. The second half of the book provides the answers, together with teaching notes and a marking scheme. There is no index but the contents list will direct you to the appropriate organ system.

In the history and counselling stations, you are advised to work with one to two colleagues to act as 'patient' and 'examiner'. The Introduction provides the background required to direct your enquiry or your counselling. Take a history from the 'patient', who will answer your questions using the history provided. The 'examiner' will mark your answers, using the scoring system outlines below, and ensure that the station is concluded in the allotted time.

The clinical examination stations include clinical photographs and test clinical skills which can be practised on appropriate patients on the ward. As the practical skills of examination cannot be assessed by a text book, a check list is included, indicating what the examiner is looking for in your examination of each system. The radiographic questions may be self-assessed by turning to the answer section.

Stations with radiographs or photographs may also carry statements requiring a 'true' or 'false' response. This adds variety to the station format and requires you to assess the answers given with respect to the radiograph or photograph. Similarly, stations with tables depicting clinical scenarios or treatment regimes test your knowledge in rearranging the latter to fit the disease.

At the back of the book there is a section that explains the marking schedule used for the stations, and a mock exam that contains five 19-station OSCE circuits: these provide typical examination scenarios.

By working through each organ system, as denoted by the chapters, you will cover most of the OSCE station scenarios and variations that you can expect to encounter in the undergraduate course.

Scoring your performance

We have chosen not to weight individual questions or items. Good is allocated 3 marks and adequate 2. In the poor/not done column the assessor can differentiate between a reasonable but inadequate mark and poor or not done. This differentiation can direct future study requirements. Each station is allocated the same mark, item scores are added in three column answers. Two of three correct responses or a mean score of 2 is a pass. A 60% correct response rate is required in two column answers. In the mock examinations two-thirds of stations should be passed to pass the examination.

Glossary

A-level	Advanced Level General Certificate of Education – School leaving Examination
ABGs	Arterial blood gases
AC	Abdominal circumference
ACE inhibitors	Angiotensin converting enzyme
ACTH	Adrenocorticotrophic hormone
Ach	Acetylcholine
ACS	Acute coronary syndrome
ADH	Anti-diuretic hormone
ADL	Activity of daily living
AF	Atrial fibrilation
AFP	Alpha-fetoprotein
aGBM	Anti-glomerular basement membrane
AGT	Angiotensin
AIDS	Acquired immune deficiency syndrome
AKA	Also known as
Alb	Albumin
Alk phos	Alkaline phosphatase
ALT	Alanine amino-transferase
AMA	Antimitochondrial antibody
ANCA	Anti neutrophil cytoplasmic antibody
Anti dsDNA	Double stranded deoxyribonucleic acid
Anti-Jo	Specific antigen
Anti-La	Specific antigen
Anti-RNP	Ribonucleic protein
Anti-Ro	Specific antigen
Anti-SCL70	Specific antigen
AP	Antero-posterior
APC gene	adenomatosis polyposis coli
APTT	Activated partial thromboplastin time
ARDS	Adult respiratory distress syndrome
ARM	Artificial rupture of membranes
AS	Aortic stenosis
ASH	Action on smoking and health
ASMA	anti- smooth muscle antibody
ASO(T)	Anti streptolysin-O-titre
AST	Aspartate amino-transferase
ATLS	Advanced trauma life support
AV	Arterio-venous

AV	Atrio-ventricular
aVF	Augmented voltage lead left lower leg
aVL	Augmented voltage lead left arm
aVR	Augmented voltage lead right arm
AVSD	Atrioventricular septal defect
AXR	Abdominal X-ray
AZT	Azidothymidine (Generic Name: Zidovudine)
BAL	Broncho-alveolar lavage
BBB	Bundle branch block
BCC	Basal cell carcinoma
BCG	Bacille Calmette-Guerin
b.d.	Bis die (twice daily)
BE	Base excess
BHL	Bilateral hilar lymphadenopathy
BMA	British Medical Association
BM stix	Blood monitoring
BM	Bone marrow
BMI	Body mass index
BMR	Basal metabolic rate
BP	Blood pressure
Bpm	Beats per minute
BRCA	Breast cancer susceptibility genes
C	Cervical
Ca	Cancer
CA	Cyclic AMP
$Ca2+$	Calcium
CAGE questionnaire	Cut down Annoyed Guilty Eye-opener
CANCA	Anti-neutrophil cytoplasmic antibody
CAPD	Chronic ambulatory peritoneal dialysis
CCa^{2+}	Corrected calcium
CD4	A surface antigen principally found on helper-inducer T-lymphocyte
CEA	Carcinoembryonic antigen
CEMD	Confidential Enquiry into Maternal Health
CESDI	Confidential Enquiry into Stillbirths and Deaths in Infancy
CF	Cystic fibrosis
CIN I II III	Cervical intraepithelial neoplasia
CK	Creatinine phosphokinase
Cl	Chloride
CLL	Chronic lymphocytic leukaemia
Cm	centimetre
CML	Chronic myeloid leukaemia

CMV	Cytomegalovirus
CNS	Central nervous system
CO2	Carbon dioxide
COCP	Combined oral contraceptive pill
COMT	Catechol O-methyl transferase
CPN	Community psychiatric nurse
CPR	Cardio pulmonary resuscitation
Cr	Creatinine
CREST	Crest syndrome – calcinosis; Raynaud's; oesophageal dysmotility; sclerodactyly; telangiectasia
CS	Caesarean section
CSF	Cerebro-spinal fluid
CSU	Catheter specimen of urine
CT	Computerised tomography
CTG	Cardiotocography
CVA	Cerebro-vascular accident
CVP	Central venous pressure
CVS	Chorionic villi sampling
CWD	Consistent with dates
CXR	Chest radiograph
DDAVP	Desmopressin, synthetic vasopressin
DIC	Disseminated intravascular coagulopathy
DIP joints	Distal inter-phalangeal joints
DKA	Diabetic keto-acidosis
dl	Decilitres
DM	Diabetes mellitus
DMSA	Dimercaptosuccinic acid
DNA	Deoxyribonucleic acid
DTP	Diphtheria-tetanus pertussis (vaccine)
DU	Duodenal ulcer
DVT	Deep vein thrombosis
DVLA	Driving vehicle licensing authority
ECG	Electrocardiogram
EEG	Electroencephalogram
EMQ	Extended matching question
ENT	Ear, nose and throat
ERCP	Endoscopic retrograde cholangiopancreatography
ESR	Erythrocyte sedimentation rate
ETEC	Enterotoxigenic Escherichia coli
EUA	Examination under anaesthesia
FBC	Full blood count
FEV1	Forced expiratory volume in one second

FFP	Fresh frozen plasma
FH	Family history
5-FU	5-Fluoro-uracil
5HT	5-hydroxy-tryptamine
fl	Femtolitres
F:M	Female:male (ratio)
FNA	Fine needle aspirate
FPC	Family planning clinic
FSH	Follicular stimulating hormone
fT4	Free thyroxine
FVC	Forced vital capacity
GABA	Gamma- amino butyric acid
GCS	Glasgow coma score
GCSE	General Certificate of Secondary Education
GCSF	Granulocyte colony stimulating factor
GDM	Gestational diabetes mellitus
GI	Gastrointestinal
GIT	Gastrointestinal tract
GMC	General Medical Council
GnRH	Gonadotrophin-releasing hormone
GP	General Practitioner
GPI	General paralysis of the insane
G6PD	Glucosa 6 phosphate dehydrogenase
GTN	Glyceryl trinitrate
GIIb/IIIa	Glycoprotein IIb/IIIa (receptor)
GU	Genito-urinary
GUM	Genito-urinary medicine
Hb	Haemoglobin
HB Alc	Glycosylated haemoglobin
HBV	Hepatitis B virus
HCG	Human chorionic gonadotrophin
HCO3−	Bicarbonate
Hct−	Haematocrit
HCV	Hepatitis C virus
HDL	High density lipoprotein
HELLP	Elevated liver enzymes and low platelet count
HIB	*Haemophilus influenzae* type B (vaccine)
HIV	Human immunodeficiency virus
HLA	Human leucocyte antigen
HONK	Hyper-osmolar non-ketotic (coma)
HR	Heart rate
HRT	Hormaone replacement therapy

HSV	Herpes simplex virus
IBD	Inflammatory bowel disease
ICP	Intra-cranial pressure
IDDM	Insulin dependent diabetes mellitus
Ig	Immunoglobulin
IgM	Immunoglobulin M
IGT	Impaired glucose tolerance
IHD	Ischaemic heart disease
Im	Intramuscular
IMB	Intermenstrual bleeding
INR	International ratio
IOL	Induction of labour
IQ	Intelligence quotient
ISMN	Iso-sorbide mono-nitrate
ITU	Intensive therapy unit
IUCD	Intrauterine contraceptive device
IUGR	Intrauterine growth retardation
IV	Intravenous
IVP	Intravenous pyelogram
IVF	Invitro fertilisation
IVU	Intravenous urogram
K^+	Potassium
Kg	Kilogramme
KPa	Kilopascals
KUB	Kidneys/ureters/bladder
L	Litre
LDL	Low density lipoprotein
LFT	Liver function tests
LGV	Lymphogranuloma venereum
LH	Luteinising hormone
LHRH	Luteinising hormone releasing hormone
LKM-1	Liver, kidney, Muscle
LLETZ	Large Loop Excision of the Transformation Zone
LMN	Lower motor neurone
LMW	Low molecular weight
LNMP	Last normal menstrual period
LSCS	Lower segment caesarean section
MAOI	Mono-amine oxidase inhibitor
MCH	Mean corpuscular haemoglobin
MCP	Meta-carpophalangeal
MCV	Mean corpuscular volume
$Mg++$	Magnesium

MI	Myocardial infarction
mmol	millimoles
MMR	Measles-mumps-rubella (vaccine)
MMSE	Mini mental state examination
Mph	miles per hour
MRI	Magnetic resonance imaging
MS	Multiple sclerosis or Mitral stenosis
MSU	Mid stream urine
Na^+	Sodium
NAD	No abnormality detected
NEC	Necrotising enterocolitis
Neut	Neutrophilis
NG	Neoplasia (new growth)
NHL	Non-Hodgkin's lymphoma
NIDDM	Non insulin dependent diabetes mellitus
NSAID	Non steroidal anti-inflammatory drug
NSU	Non-specific urethritis
O2	Oxygen
OA	Osteoarthritis
OCP	oral contraceptive pill
Od	omni die (once daily)
OGD	Oesophagogastroduodenoscopy
OSCE	Objective structured clinical examination
PA	Postero-anterior
$PaCO_2$	arterial pressure of carbon dioxide
PaO_2	arterial pressure of oxygen
PAN	Perinuclear anti-neutrophilic
Panca	Perinuclear anti-neutrophilic cytoplasmic antibody
PCO	Polycystic ovaries
PCOS	Polycystic ovary syndrome
PCP	Pneumocystis carinii pneumonia
PCR	Polymerase chain reaction
PCV	Packed cell volume
PDA	Patent ductus arteriosus
PE	Pulmonary embolism
PEA	Persistent electrical activity
PEFR	Peak expiratory flow rate
PET	positron emission tomography
pH	Puissance d'Hydrogen = $- \log (H+)$
PICU	Paediatric intensive care unit
PID	Pelvic inflammatory disease
Plats	Platelets

PMH	Previous medical history
PND	Paroxysmal nocturnal dyspnoea
PNS	Peripheral nervous system
PO4⁻	Phosphate
PPH	Post partum haemorrhage
PPI	Proton pump inhibitor
PR	Per rectum
PRHO	Pre-registration house officer
PRN	Pro re nata (as required)
PSA	Prostatic specific antigen
PT	Prothrombin time
PV	Per vagina
RBC	Red blood count
RCT	Randomised, controlled trial
Retics	Reticulocytes
ROM	Range of movement
RTA	Road traffic accident
RTA (I–IV)	Renal tubular acidosis
SACD	Subacute combined degeneration of the spinal cord
SAH	Subarachnoid haemorrhage
SARS	Severe acute respiratory syndrome
SCC	Squamous cell carcinoma
SDH	Subdural haemorrhage
SHBG	Sex hormone binding globulin
SIADH	Syndrome of inappropriate antidiuretic hormone secretion
SLE	Systemic lupus erythema
SOL	Space occupying lesion
SROM	spontaneous rupture of membranes
SSRI	Selective serotonin reuptake inhibitors
STEMI	ST elevation MI
STI	Sexually transmitted disease
Substance P	Vasoactive peptide and sensory neurotransmitter found in nerve cells and specialist gut endocrine cells SVT Supraventricular tachycardia
SVD	Spontaneous vaginal delivery
SVT	Supraventricular tachycardia
SXR	Skull X-ray
T3	Tri-iodo – thyronine
T4	Tetra – iodo -thyronine (thyroxine)
TB	Tuberculosis
TBM	Tuberculous meningitis
Tds	Ter die sumendus – (to be taken three times daily)

TED	Thrombo-embolic
TFTs	Thyroid function tests
T Helper	Thymus (lymphocytes)
TKco	Transfer coefficient
TIA	Transient ischaemic attack
TOP	Termination of pregnancy
TPA	Tissue plasminogen activator
TPHA	Treponema pallidum haemagglutination assay
TSH	Thyroid stimulating hormone
TT	Thrombin time
TVM	Transvaginal monitoring
U&Es	Urea and electrolytes
UMN	Upper motor neurone
Ur	Urea
USS	Ultrasound scan
UTI	Urinary tract infection
UV	Ultra violet
UV prolapse	Utero-vaginal prolapse
VDRL	Venereal disease research laboratory
VMA	Vanillylmandelic acid
V/Q scan	Ventilation/perfusion scan
VSD	Ventricular septal defect
V-V Fistula	Vesico-vaginal fistula
VZV	Varicella zoster virus
WCC	White cell count

Normal Values

In the majority of OSCE data interpretation stations it is customary in undergraduate examination to provide a set of normal values. Please refer to the list below when attempting any of the data interpretation stations in all three volumes of OSCEs.

Haematology

Haemoglobin		
	Males	13.5 – 17.5 g/dl
	Females	11.5 – 15.5 g/dl
MCV		76 – 98 fl
PCV		35 – 55%
WCC		$4 - 11 \times 10^9/l$
Neut.		$2.5 - 7.58 \times 10^9/l$
Lymph.		$1.5 - 3.5 \times 10^9/l$
Plt		$150 - 400 \times 10^9/l$
ESR		0 – 10 mm in the 1st hour
PT		10.6 – 14.9 s
PTT		23.0 – 35.0 s
TT		10.5 – 15.5 s
Fib		125 – 300 mg/dl
Vitamin B_{12}		160 – 900 pmol/l
Folate		1.5 µg/l
Ferritin		
	Males	20 – 250 µmol/l
	Females	10 – 120 µmol/l

Immunoglobulins

IgM	0.5 – 2.0 g/l
IgG	5 – 16 g/l
IgA	1.0 – 4.0 g/l

Biochemistry

Na^+	135 – 145 mmol/l
K^+	3.5 – 5.0 mmol/l
Urea (ur)	2.5 – 6.5 mmol/l
Cr	50 – 120 µmol/l
ALT	5 – 30 iu/l
AST	10 – 40 iu/l
Bili.	2 – 17 µmol/l
Alk Phos	30 – 130 iu/l
Albumin	35 – 55 g/l
γGT	5 – 30 iu/l

αFP	< 10 ku/l
CCA[2]	2.20 – 2.60 mmol/l
PO_4^{2-}	0.70 – 1.40 mmol/l
CK	23 – 175 iu/l
LDH	100 – 190 iu/l
Amylase	< 200 u/l
Lactate	0.5 – 2.2 mmol/l
Mg^{2+}	0.75 – 1.00 mmol/l
Urate	0.1 – 0.4 mol/l
CRP	0 – 10 mg/l

Diabetes

Glucose		
	Random	3.5 – 5.5 mmol/l*
	Fasting	< 7 mmol/l
HbA1c		< 7.0%

Endocrinology

TSH		0.17 – 3.2 mu/l
fT_4		11 – 22 pmol/l
fT_3		3.5 – 5 pmol/l
Cortisol		
	0900	140 – 500 nmol/l
	2400	50 – 300 nmol/l
Growth hormone		< 10 ng/ml
Cholesterol		< 5.2 mmol/l
Triglycerides		0 – 1.5 mmol/l
LDL		< 3.5 mmol/l
HDL		> 1.0 mmol/l
Total/ HDL		< 5.0
FSH		1 – 25 u/l
LH		1 – 70 u/l
Prolactin		< 400 mu/l

Blood gases

pH	7.35 – 7.45
pA (CO_2)	4.6 – 6.0 kPa
pA (CO_2)	10.5 – 13.5 kPa
HCO_3^- (bicarbonate)	24 – 30 mmol/l
BE	–2 – 2.0 mmol/l

CSF

Protein	< 0.45 g/l
Glucose	2.5 – 3.9 mmol/l (two-thirds plasma)
Cells	< 5 (WCC)
Opening pressure	6 – 20 cmH$_2$O
* If >5.5 then OGTT 2 h:	7 – 11.1 = IGT
	> 11.1 = DM

Generic approach to Examinations

As with all OSCE stations, clinical examination stations should have clear, precise candidate instructions. **Read them carefully before starting** (and before asking any questions!) and if you are still unclear as to what you are being asked to do, clarify the task with the examiner.

For all clinical examinations you should try and follow the five steps given below. Some examinations may require you to modify or vary these stages:

1 **Introduction and consent**
2 **Observation and comment**
3 **Palpation**
4 **Auscultation**
5 **Presentation of findings and differential diagnoses or causes**

1 Introduction and consent

- Introduce yourself to the patient: with your name and role
- Explain what you would like to do and obtain verbal consent for the examination, eg 'I am just going to listen to your heart sounds, 'is that alright?' or 'Would it be alright if I examine your chest, legs'
- Keep these requests simple and in lay terms. Avoid medical jargon such as 'I would like to examine your peripheral nervous system' or 'would it be alright if I examine your cranial nerves?' Better to ask 'Would it be alright if I examine the function of your arms or legs' or ' Would it be alright if I examine the function of the nerves that control your face?'

2 Observation and comment

- Stand at the **END** of the patient's bed and comment on relative positives and negative manifestations. Look for relevant signs and they will be there – If you fail to look for them, they may not appear!
- Do not just say 'I'm looking for...'. **Comment** on the presence or absence of relevant signs
- Move back to the patient's right-hand side, re-clarify before starting your examination if you should start at the hands (if not stated in the instructions)
- **Look** for relevant signs – **comment** on their presence/absence.
- BUT expect to be challenged on findings/causes of anything you mention.

3 Palpation

- Be sure you have washed your hands in warm water before commencing any the examination. There is usually an alcohol wash at the bedside of each patient, which you should use between stations. If not, you should wash your hands between each patient, but be careful you do not leave the examiner behind, as he or she might be a little irritated.
- Whenever palpating:
  - (i)   Reassure the patient before starting
  - (ii)   Watch the patient's face for distress at all times
  - (iii) Apologise if any distress is caused
  - (iv) If distressed before the start of the examination – suggest appropriate analgesia.

4 Auscultation

- Understand what the stethoscope and its components are for, ie how to use the bell and the diaphragm (Bell = Low frequency) and even which way round to put the earpieces in your ears!
- Always tap the piece (bell or diaphragm) you are about to place on the patient with a finger, thus ensuring it is orientated the correct way. This saves 'no sounds heard': embarrassing silence!
- Always make sure the stethoscope pieces are warm (like you hands) before placing them on the patient.
- Your stethoscope should hang so the bell/diaphragm lies just below your waistline. This means you may need to cut longer tubes down but be wary of cutting off too much!
- With the more expensive/sophisticated stethoscopes you will hear sounds more easily and clearly. However, you may wish to buy a mid range one first to learn the basics.
- Know how to use the stethoscope, if you choose to buy an expensive/sophisticated one.

As with all the examination techniques, palpation, ballotting, auscultation and percussion, practice makes perfect! Initially you may feel more comfortable practising in the clinical skills laboratory on manikins and normal people, however **you must** practice in the various clinical settings on patients with and without clinical signs. Essential parts of the examination cannot be practised on friends and mannequins. Overcoming embarrassment or anxieties, talking and interacting with patients and relatives and, most importantly, recognising when patients are ill and eliciting clinical signs. At the end of every examination make sure you cover the patient up and thank them. Take every opportunity to examine patients, checking appropriate subjects with housemen and your peers, but make sure you have permission from the patient and the sister-in-charge.

5 Presentation of clinical findings, differential diagnoses and causes.

- Your presentation should be simple and concise. Present relevant positives and negatives, a differential diagnosis or causes.
- If you know the diagnosis, present the positive findings to support your diagnosis.
- 'This well looking, middle-aged man has signs consistent with aortic stenosis as evidenced by his low volume pulse which was slow rising in character. He has a narrow pulse pressure and his apex beat is hyperdynamic but undisplaced. On auscultation he has a grade 4/6 ejection systolic murmur heard loudest in the aortic area and radiating to the carotids. He has no signs of heart failure and no stigmata of endocarditis'.
- If you do not know the diagnosis, present the relevant positive and negative findings in a concise, logical manner. The simplest way to achieve this is to present the evaluations in the order of your examination, ie start at the hands, work up the forearm, the arm (including blood pressure), the face and neck, chest, abdomen and other regions of interest.
- 'This well looking middle-aged man had no peripheral stigmata of cardiovascular disease. His pulse was 72 bpm and regular, it was symmetrical and I was unsure but I think the character was abnormal. His blood pressure was 110/100 but I couldn't see his jugular venous pulse. His carotids were easily felt and had an abnormal character, although I couldn't define it. The apex beat was undisplaced and forceful. He had no heaves or thrills. On auscultation he had a systolic murmur heard loudest in the aortic area and I think it radiated to the carotids and the mitral area. He had no pulmonary or peripheral oedema. In summary, I think he may have aortic stenosis'.
- At the end of your presentation you should present a list of the common differentials or causes of the patient's problem.
- The examiner may challenge you on anything that you state, eg if you say the patient has clubbing, you might be asked some causes of clubbing.
- As with all clinical skills, presentation of findings and differentials requires practice.

Chapter 1:
Cardiovascular Diseases
and Haematology

Contents

CHAPTER 1

Cardiovascular Diseases and Haematology

Cardiovascular History

Chest pain

This is one of the most common presenting symptoms that a doctor will come across and it is, therefore, very important to try to differentiate the causes from the history. All causes of chest pain must be defined by:

- **Character**
  Dull, sharp, severe, pleuritic, burning
  Common descriptions – 'like a knife'; 'like a weight on my chest'
- **Site**
  Retrosternal, anterior, unilateral, can it be defined by one point on the chest wall?
- **Radiation**
  To the upper limbs, the neck, the jaw
  Epigastric – inferior ischaemic cardiac pain
  Interscapular/back – dissecting thoracic aortic aneurysm, posterior cardiac pain
- **Exacerbating factors**
  Exertion – need to define exercise tolerance in minutes or metres
  Respiration – pain worse with inspiration implies pleuritic pain
  Coughing/movement of the chest wall – pleuritic or musculoskeletal
- **Relieving factors**
  Stopping any exertion
  Glyceryl trinitrate (GTN) spray or tablets
  Oxygen – often given by paramedics in the ambulance
  NSAIDs
- **Associated factors**
  Nausea and vomiting
  Shortness of breath
  Clamminess/sweating
  Dizziness/faint
  Loss of consciousness

Palpitations
Haemoptysis, cough, sputum
Recent chest wall trauma

Differential diagnoses

- Ischaemic cardiac chest pain, angina or myocardial infarction
- Pericarditis: sharp, anterior chest pain, relieved with sitting forward, worse on lying down
- Myocarditis: may be angina or pericarditis type pain
- Musculoskeletal chest pain: variable in characteristics, depends on the cause
- Pleuritic pain: worse with inspiration and coughing, patient can often define the exact location on the chest wall by pointing with one finger
- Costochondral pain: worse with pressure over the costochondral joints, coughing and movements of the chest wall (viral costochondritis is eponymously known as Tietze's syndrome)

Dyspnoea or shortness of breath

Associated with:

- Exertion: define exercise tolerance (walking) in minutes or metres; exertion may be limited to activities of daily living (eg washing or transferring between pieces of furniture) if dyspnoea is severe
- Cough, sputum, haemoptysis
- Wheeze
- Peripheral oedema

Paroxysmal nocturnal dyspnoea (PND)

This is a manifestation of heart failure; the patient describes waking feeling short of breath. The feeling is relieved by sitting up, sitting on the edge of the bed or getting up out of bed.

Orthopnoea

This is the sensation of breathlessness on lying flat. It should be defined by the number of pillows that the patient sleeps with. Patients with extreme orthopnoea will often sleep in a chair or sitting upright in bed as they are unable to lie down at all.

Peripheral oedema

- Swelling of the ankles, calves and thighs
- Ascites, pleural effusion

Differential diagnoses

- Renal failure/nephrotic syndrome
- Hepatic failure

Palpitations

- Defined as fast or slow; regular or irregular
- The patient should be asked to beat out the palpitations on the table or bed
- 'Sinister' symptoms associated with palpitations: dizziness, loss of consciousness, nausea, sweating/clamminess and dyspnoea

These symptoms may be the result of either haemodynamic compromise or are due to associated autonomic changes. Patients often describe a feeling of 'being aware of their heart beat in bed or whilst sitting quietly'. Unless this is associated with any of the symptoms above, it is normal and the patient may be reassured.

Cardiovascular Examination

- Introduce yourself; explain the examination and gain verbal consent to proceed
- Ensure the patient is comfortable, correctly positioned at 45° and adequately exposed. On observation from the end of the bed – comment on the wellbeing of the patient ie are they well or unwell, then from the:
  - Feet – peripheral oedema, signs of PVD, scar of saphenous vein graft harvest, ulceration, amputations (toes, feet, BKA)
  - Abdomen – ascites, aortic aneurysm, femoral-popliteal by-pass scars
  - Chest – sternotomy and lateral thoracotomy scars, chest deformity, permanent pacemaker

> **If a sternotomy scar is present listen for the 'crocodile sign' – metallic valves will often be audible from the end of the bed and 'tick' like the alarm clock inside the crocodile in *Peter Pan***

  - Neck – jugular venous pulse and carotid pulsation
  - Face – anaemia, mitral facies, peri-orbital xanthelasma

Return to the patient. Assess and comment on:

Hands
- Stigmata of endocarditis (Janeway lesions, Osler's nodes, splinter haemorrhages)
- Clubbing; cyanosis; anaemia; tar staining; vasculitic changes and signs of PVD

Radial pulse *– time for 15 seconds – (thus all pulses must be a multiple of four since 15 × 4 = 60 seconds or beats per minute). During these 15 seconds assess and comment on the **rate, rhythm or regularity, volume, and symmetry and vessel wall.***

Ask the patient 'Do you have pain in shoulder – if No, raise the right forearm up above the level of the right shoulder (thus above the heart) whilst palpating for a collapsing pulse. (This is a sign of aortic regurgitation.)

Ask the examiner – 'I'd now like to know the blood pressure' – Do not ignore the answer! Consider: *is it high, low or normal, is there a normal pulse pressure (the difference between systolic and diastolic pressure; normal = 120–80 = 40 mmHg).*

Face
- Eyes – assess for anaemia, corneal arcus, xanthelasma
- Mitral facies
- Mouth – anaemia, central cyanosis (associated with cor pulmonale)

Neck
- Assess the jugular venour pulse (JVP) with the patient sat at 45° (see JVP station)
- Carotid pulse – assess the character, the symmetry (but never feel both carotids simultaneously!) and for the presence of bruits

Praecordium
- Re-examine for sternotomy and lateral thoracotomy (valvuloplasty) scars
  Palpate:
  - **Apex beat** (define position and character).
  - **Left parasternal heave**.
  - **Thrills** (palpable murmurs) – if present they need to be timed with the cardiac cycle, ie diastolic or systolic

Auscultate

By trying to put the signs together as you examine, you should have an idea of what you are going to hear on auscultation.

> **Listen for it – and you will hear it**
> **('Seek and ye shall find')**

Eg consider the following signs
1 A low volume pulse, atrial fibrillation, mitral facies, an undisplaced/'tapping' apex beat. These are the signs of mitral stenosis. So as you take out your stethoscope which murmur are you trying to hear?

Answer – A low pitched rumbling mid-diastolic murmur heard loudest at the apex with the bell of the stethoscope.

2 A low volume pulse, narrow pulse pressure, slow rising carotid pulse, sustained/ undisplaced apex beat. These are the signs of aortic stenosis. What murmur will you be straining to hear?

Answer – An ejection systolic murmur, heard loudest in the aortic area, radiating to the carotids.

Ensure:

1 You know and listen in all four areas of the heart.

2 Lean the patient on their left. Listen specifically for mitral stenosis with the bell. It is a low, rumbling, mid-diastolic murmur (MDM) heard loudest at the apex. Listen with the diaphragm for the pan-systolic murmur (PSM) of mitral regurgitation – this is often a 'blowing' murmur radiating to the axilla.

3 Reposition patient back at 45°/facing forward.

4 Listen in the tricuspid and pulmonary regions with the diaphragm.

5 Listen for the ejection systolic murmur (ESM) of aortic stenosis which radiates to the carotids.

6 Now listen with the diaphragm at the lower left sternal edge with the patient leaning forward in expiration. (This is for the early diastolic murmur (EDM) of aortic regurgitation).

NB – Left side murmurs get louder with expiration. Right side murmurs get louder with inspiration.

- Whilst the patient is leaning forward listen at the lung bases for pulmonary oedema. Feel for sacral oedema.
- Reposition the patient so the they are sitting back comfortably at 45°.
- Cover the patient with blanket or bed clothes.
- Thank the patient and ensure they are comfortable and not distressed.

Now turn to examiner and present the positive and relevant negative findings, the diagnosis and differentials. You may be asked about complications, investigations and management of any given diagnosis.

Peripheral Vascular Disease

In the UK vascular disease is produced by atherosclerosis in over 90% of cases. Coronary artery disease accounts for more than 40% and cerebrovascular disease, more than 10% of deaths and considerable disability. Lower limb disease usually presents with intermittent claudication (calf pain on exercise) and in 8 – 10% of patients this progresses to rest pain and gangrene. The latter symptoms and disabling claudication may require therapeutic intervention and even amputation.

In the history, these three areas must be assessed, together with questions related to gut and renal ischaemia and associated risk factors, particularly smoking, diabetes and hypertension. There is also an increased instance of vascular disease in obesity, lipid disorders and often a family history.

You may be asked to examine lower limb pulses in a claudicant or a model, or to assess pulses and the nutritional status of the limb in more advanced ischaemia, when the examiner will indicate whether the examination should include the whole of the cardiovascular system.

Examination of the lower limbs in peripheral vascular disease

In the lower limb, pulses must be examined, the patient, wearing underclothes, lies flat on the bed with one pillow under their head and both legs exposed over their full length, removing all bed clothes and bed cradles.

An artery is pressed backwards on an underlying bony surface, its diameter and the status of its wall are assessed. The degree of pulsation, any enlargement, and the rate, rhythm, character and the volume of the pulse are compared with the same features of the radial pulse. The femoral artery is compressed onto the head of the femur, this is in the mid-inguinal point (midway between the anterior superior iliac spine and the symphysis pubis). Both sides are compared and comment on the regularity, volumes and symmetry, and the state of the vessel wall.

Examine the popliteal pulses individually and then compare them. Compress the distal popliteal onto the back of the upper end of the tibia with the tips of the fingers from both hands wrapped around the upper leg, compressing between the heads of gastrocnemius. The subject's leg may be slightly flexed and the foot placed on the bed. It is easy to do this sitting on the bed (Sister not usually being present to contest this habit!).

The dorsalis pedis artery commences midway between the two malleoli and extends towards the first digital web. It is best palpated over the proximal metatarsals, lateral to the head of flexor hallucis longus in this line.

The posterior tibial artery passes into the sole midway between the medial malleolus and the medial prominence of the heel. It is compressed onto the medial side of the talus at this point.

A perforating peroneal artery may be palpated just anterior to the lateral malleolus. This is looked for after the previous two pulses, particularly if they are weak or absent (either congenitally or as the result of disease).

Place a stethoscope over both femoral arteries, and the adductor hiatus on the medial aspect of both thighs, a hand's breadth above the knee, for bruits; disease is common in both these areas.

Observe the nutritional status of the limb in ischaemia. The skin over the foot and lower leg is thin with loss of subcutaneous tissue. There is pallor, due to low perfusion and this can be accentuated by lifting the heel off the bed. In severe ischaemia, forward perfusion is determined by the extent that the veins empty and leave a gutter (venous guttering). The point at which this happens is called Berger's angle. If the limb is retained for at least a minute in this position, it goes very pale; after this has happened, ask the patient to sit on the side of the bed with the legs dependent. The veins rapidly or slowly refill from the toes upwards and the colour returns. There is usually a period of reactive hyperaemia, when the limb goes brightly red-purple. The length of time taken for venous filling and for the reactive hyperaemia should be noted. In severe ischaemia this is often 40 seconds and 3 minutes respectively.

In severe ischaemia, there may be a break in skin continuity, such as a pressure sore over either malleolus, the heel or the side of the foot, or ulceration of the webs or over the tips of the toes. This progresses to gangrene of the toes and more proximally, as the severity of the disease increases.

You must be able to describe the presence, the site and colour changes of ulceration, with its size, shape and edge; the latter is usually punched out with exposed underlying tendon, ligaments and bone, with a variable degree of gangrenous changes. When there is associated diabetes, there may also be inflammation and induration, with deep suppuration of tendon sheaths and joints, together with a variable degree of gangrenous changes.

Venous disease

1 Varicose veins

Varicose veins are thin-walled, tortuous, dilated and lengthened, with incompetent valves. The incompetence may be primary, often with a family history, or secondary to deep venous thrombosis. On rare occasions the veins are part of a congenital vascular malformation or an acquired arteriovenous fistula. Incompetence gives rise to venous hypertension when standing, and this increases tissue fluid, with swelling and subsequent trophic skin changes. The latter are due to poor skin nutrition with slow healing of any minor trauma and, eventually, ulceration.

Symptoms are very variable, often worse in warm weather and during pregnancy. In the history it should be established whether the veins are primary, starting in the teens with a family history, or postphlebitic with or without anticoagulation treatment. The presenting problem is often cosmetic, and there may be aching, particularly at the end of the day, after prolonged standing with heaviness, cramps and swelling. Note symptoms of eczema, itching, pigmentation, bleeding or chronic ulceration.

On examination note the distribution of the veins; long saphenous varices outnumber short saphenous by about seven to one. There may be skin changes of eczema, pigmentation or ulceration. The features of ulceration and the differential diagnoses are considered in Station 1.11. Look and feel for cough impulses over the saphenofemoral and the saphenopopliteal junctions, and see if there is a propagated tap impulse distally along a length of abnormal vein, denoting incompetence.

The use of a tourniquet at sites along a limb, after emptying the veins, indicates where dependent filling can be controlled or whether there is leaking of blood from the deep to superficial veins, through incompetent perforators below the level of the tourniquet.

Apply a below-knee venous tourniquet and ask the patient to stand on tip-toe ten times. If the deep veins are blocked the muscle pump forces blood into the superficial varices, whereas, with normal deep veins, the pump empties the superficial system. The use of a Doppler ultrasonic probe is an effective means of identifying reversal of the superficial venous flow, incompetent perforators and abnormalities of the deep system.

2 Deep venous thrombosis (DVT)

Thrombosis is characteristically attributed to Virchow's triad of venous stasis, coaguable states and endothelial injury; however it is usually due to more than one of these contributing factors. A number of conditions predispose to this problem; they include trauma, operative procedures, particularly of the hip joint, pregnancy and female gender, ageing (> 40), obesity, malignancy and previous DVT. The most common site of origin of a DVT is in the soleal plexus of the calf. Propagation occurs into the popliteal, femoral and, occasionally, iliac veins. Symptomatically DVT may go unnoticed but suspicion should be raised by any leg pain or swelling in patients at risk, particularly in the post-operative period.

In patients with no identifiable risk, a procoagulant or thrombophilia screen should be undertaken. This should include FBC, INR, APPT, Protein C and S levels, factor V Leiden and anti-cardiolipin antibody.

On examination there may be a low grade pyrexia and swelling. Tenderness in the calf and along the length of the lower limb veins may be slight or marked and, in extreme cases, result in venous gangrene. However, the signs, like the symptoms, may be minimal, requiring careful examination for traces of peripheral oedema, and palpation of the length of the calf and popliteal fossa, and along the anteromedial thigh, for tenderness. The diagnosis can usually be confirmed by ultrasonic Doppler scanning.

The clinical importance of DVT is the danger of pulmonary embolism during the developing phase and the late sequelae of the post-phlebitic syndrome (see Station 1.11 regarding ulcers). For this reason prophylactic subcutaneous heparin is prescribed in high-risk patients with anti-embolic compression stockings; proven DVT is treated with full anticoagulation.

STATION 1.1 *(Answers – page 157)*

History

You are a house officer attached to a general medical firm. The registrar has asked you to take a history from a 43-year-old man with chest pain who has been referred by the casualty officer. Please take a history of the presenting complaint and any other relevant history with a view to making a diagnosis.

(5 minute station)

STATION 1.2

History

You are a medical student attached to a general medical firm. You have been asked by the SHO on call to take a history from a 29-year-old man complaining of chest pain. Please take a history of the presenting complaint and any other relevant history with a view to making a diagnosis.

(5 minute station)

STATION 1.3

History: Preparatory

Please use the next five minutes to read the information below. You may then proceed to Station 1.3a.

You are a GP. The next patient is a 33-year-old man, who has asked to see you because he is worried about some chest pains he has been experiencing lately. His father died six weeks ago of a myocardial infarction, aged 62 years old, and he is worried he is at risk of angina. He recently went for a routine life assurance examination and investigations taken at the time are shown below.

FBC; U+Es; Glucose; TFTs – normal

Cholesterol – total 6.9; LDL 5.0; HDL 1.2

(Target total cholesterol < 5.5 mmol/l)

CXR; ECG – within normal limits

BMI – 29.5 (normal limits 22–28)

(5 minute station)

STATION 1.3a

Counselling

You are a GP. The patient referred to above has come to see you regarding the recent onset of chest pain which he is particularly worried about because of the death of his father six weeks ago of an acute MI. Please assess his chest pain and risk factors for ischaemic heart disease and counsel him with regard to any lifestyle changes you think may be necessary.

(10 minute station)

STATION 1.4

History

You are a GP. The next patient is a 67-year-old woman who has come to see you because she is having palpitations. Please take a history of the presenting complaint with a view to making a diagnosis.

(5 minute station)

STATION 1.5

History

You are a GP. The next patient is a 63-year-old man who has come to see you complaining of exertional dyspnoea. Please take a history of the presenting complaint and any relevant history with a view to making a diagnosis.

(5 minute station)

STATION 1.6

Examination

You are a medical student. The next patient has either:

1 Cardiovascular symptoms eg chest pain, exertional dyspnoea, peripheral oedema

or

2 Risks for cardiovascular disease eg heavy smoker or hypertension

Please perform a full cardiovascular examination and present your findings as you go along or at the end of your examination.

(10 minute station)

STATION 1.7

Examination

You are a medical PRHO. You have been asked to perform a cardiovascular examination on the ward round by your SpR/Consultant. Please start at assessment of the carotid pulse and continue. You do not need to examine the face or hands.

(5 minute station)

STATION 1.8

Examination

You are a junior medical student attached to a GP surgery. You have been asked by the practice nurse to repeat the BP of a patient who was found to have a BP = 150/90 at his/her initial visit earlier today. (He/she has been sitting quietly for 20 minutes.) Please assess the patient's blood pressure. The nurse may ask you to comment on any abnormalities or likely variations.

(5 minute station)

STATION 1.9

Examination

You are a senior medical student attached to a medical firm. The SpR has asked you to assess this patient's JVP. He/she will ask you some questions regarding the assessment as you proceed.

(5 minute station)

STATION 1.10

Examination

This 72-year-old patient complains of pain in his left calf and thigh on walking 30 metres on the flat.

1 Clinically assess the vascularity of the lower limbs.

2 Demonstrate how you would obtain the ankle:brachial pressure index on the symptomatic limb. Equipment provided: sphygmomanometer, hand-held Doppler machine and couch.

(5 minute station)

STATION 1.11

Examination

You are a medical student in a surgical outpatient department, when a 67-year-old lady is referred with recurrence of her leg ulcer. This has been present intermittently for over eight years.

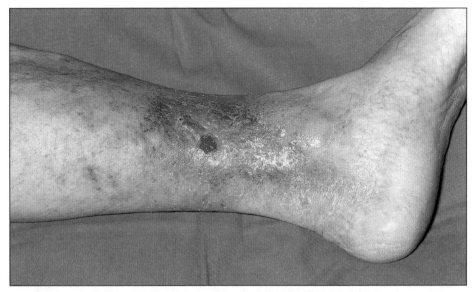

fig 1.11

Please comment on the ulcer, and state what additional symptoms and signs you must look for in this patient.

(5 minute station)

STATION 1.12

Examination

You are a medical student and the subject in the next station may be introduced as a manikin or a patient who is complaining of calf claudication after walking more than 100 metres.

Please examine the lower limb peripheral pulses in this subject/patient and tell me what you are doing as you go along.

(5 minute station)

STATION 1.13

Examination

You are a surgical PRHO on a ward round with your consultant and are asked to examine the lower limbs of a 70-year-old gentleman. He has just been admitted because he has to sleep in a chair at night, as he has severe foot pain if he goes to bed.

You have been asked to explain your findings to the medical students on the ward round. (The illustration is of the patient's left foot.)

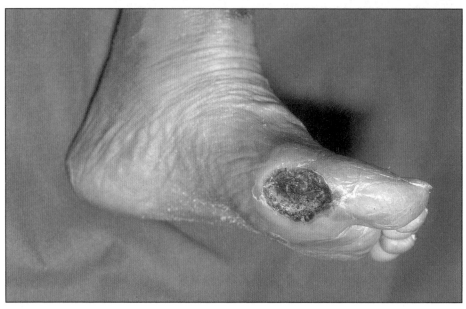

fig 1.13

(5 minute station)

STATION 1.14

Investigation

The table below lists six coagulation disorders. Please indicate the correct results of the screening tests (I, II, III) as normal, raised or lowered and identify the appropriate treatment for each of these conditions by rearranging the last column.

(5 minute station)

Coagulation disorder	I: TT	II: PT	III: APPT	IV: Treatment
1 Thrombocytopenia				A Factor VIII concentrate
2 Haemophilia				B Protamine sulphate
3 Disseminated intravascular coagulation				C Platelet concentrate
4 Patient on heparin therapy				D Fresh frozen plasma (FFP)
5 Massive transfusion of stored blood				E Phytomenadione (Vitamin K) (Synkavite) plus Factors II, IX, X and VII
6 Patient on warfarin therapy				F Whole blood, crystalloid or red cell concentrates. Treat underlying cause (eg sepsis). Plus FFP, platelet concentrates.

TT Thrombin Time
PT Prothrombin Time
APPT Activated Partial Thromoplastin Time

STATION 1.15

Investigation

All of the patients below are suffering from haemolytic anaemia.

Please match the patient histories with the correct diagnoses and markers of their disease.

Patient history	Diagnosis	Disease marker
1 29-year-old Italian man presenting with haemolytic anaemia after a meal containing fava beans	(A) Sickle cell disease	(a) Warm antibodies (IgG) Coombs' positive AIHA
2 34-year-old man with a cough, fever, bullous myringitis and erythema multiforme	(B) β-thalassaemia	(b) Hb β chains have glutamine rather than valine at position 6
3 7-year-old Greek girl with transfusion siderosis and frontal bossing of the skull	(C) G6PD deficiency	(c) Hb electrophoresis shows increased Hb F
4 A 24-year-old woman with butterfly malar rash; renal failure secondary to glomerulonephritis and anti-double stranded DNA Ig antibodies	(D) Mycoplasma pneumonia	(d) Heinz bodies in the blood
5 A 21-year-old Afrocaribbean man with abdominal and bone pain	(E) SLE	(e) Cold antibodies (IgM) Coombs' positive AIHA

(5 minute station)

Answers

1 ( ) ( )   4 ( ) ( )

2 ( ) ( )   5 ( ) ( )

3 ( ) ( )

STATION 1.16

Investigation

You are the house officer covering the routine anticoagulation clinic. The patients' current INR results are shown below. Please match the patients with the most appropriate advice.

(5 minute station)

Patient history	INR	Management advice
1 29-year-old woman with mitral valve replacement	1.9	A Stop warfarin therapy
2 21-year-old woman previously on the OCP presenting 3 weeks after admission for a right calf DVT	2.5	B Admit; omit warfarin Consider FFP if active bleeding
3 41-year-old man with known biventricular cardiac failure and atrial fibrillation	10.1	C Check compliance. Increase the dose of warfarin
4 61-year-old man on warfarin for previous thromboembolic stroke	3.5	D Omit warfarin for two days. Remind GP and patient to check the INR and the need for care with erythromycin
5 47-year-old woman with proven PE 7 months ago	2.8	E Continue same dose of warfarin
6 31-year-old man with recurrent PE, now presenting after a course of antibiotics for a chest infection	5.9	F Decrease the dose of warfarin

Answers

(1) ( )   (4) ( )

(2) ( )   (5) ( )

(3) ( )   (6) ( )

STATION 1.17

Investigation

The blood bottles shown in fig 1.17 are the standard bottles used in the NHS in the UK. Please indicate which bottle is used for the investigations listed below.

(5 minute station)

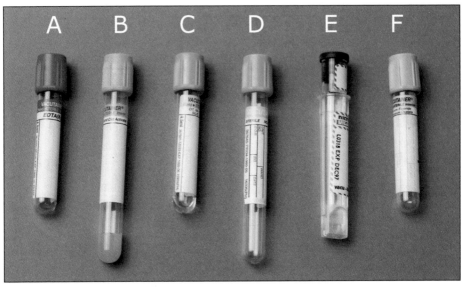

fig 1.17

Blood test	Blood bottle
1 Check Hb post transfusion	
2 Blood glucose	
3 Serum lipids	
4 Cross match	
5 Serum potassium	
6 Autoantibody screen	
7 Malaria screen	
8 Atypical pneumonia screen	
9 Thyroid function tests	
10 Platelet count – thrombocytopenia	
11 INR	
12 Amylase	
13 FDPs (fibrinogen degradation products)	
14 Serum osmolality	
15 ESR	

STATION 1.18

Investigation

The patients below have all been found to have a raised serum creatine phosphokinase (CPK). Please match the patient history with the correct diagnosis.

(5 minute station)

Patient history	Diagnosis
1 A 27-year-old schizophrenic man recently started on droperidol, now presents with muscle rigidity and pyrexial illness	(A) Anterior myocardial infarction
2 A 69-year-old woman with bilateral subdural haemorrhages on CT head scan	(B) Simvastatin induced myositis
3 An endurance marathon runner admitted post 300 km race, with leg pains and renal failure	(C) Dermatomyositis
4 A 43-year-old Scottish man 6 weeks post MI now presents with proximal limb pains	(D) Neuroleptic malignant syndrome
5 A 46-year-old smoker with severe central chest pain. ECG shows ST elevation in leads V1 to V4	(E) Ecstasy overdose
6 A 52-year-old man with proximal limb wasting, a skin rash and a suspicious mass on the chest X-ray	(F) Rhabdomyolysis
7 A 17-year-old woman brought in from a 'rave party' with hyperpyrexia and muscle rigidity	(G) Recurrent falls

Answers

1 ( )   5 ( )

2 ( )   6 ( )

3 ( )   7 ( )

4 ( )

The ECG – Introduction

This section deals with how to interpret an ECG; it is by no means comprehensive and assumes the student has a basic knowledge of the ECG.

We recommend the following steps every time you read an ECG. In this way you will not miss the simple abnormalities that can be easily overlooked.

Rate

Measurement of the rate of the ECG (ie the heart rate) is determined by the speed of the machine. Always check that the ECG is running at 25 mm/second; 25 mm are equal to five large squares, therefore in one minute the paper travels (5 × 60) = 300 large squares. To ascertain the heart rate, measure between two consecutive points (eg two R waves) and divide this figure into 300. Thus, if there are four large squares between two R waves the heart rate is 75 beats per minute (bpm). Independent of the rhythm, tachycardia is defined as a rate greater than 100 bpm, and bradycardia below 60 bpm.

Rhythm

The rhythm is determined by the presence or absence of a P wave. Once you have determined the presence or absence of a P wave, you need to decide whether the rhythm is regular or irregular.

- **P wave present**
  Regular: sinus rhythm
  Irregular: sinus arrhythmia, Wenckebach
- **P wave absent**
  Regular: narrow QRS complexes
  Nodal: junctional/idioventricular
  Atrial flutter with 2:1, 3:1 block
  Broad complexes
  Ventricular tachycardia: SVT with aberrant conduction (ie bundle branch block)
  Irregular: narrow complexes – atrial fibrillation (AF)
  Atrial flutter with variable block
  Broad complexes
  Ventricular fibrillation
  AF with bundle branch block

P wave morphology

This can only be commented on if there are P waves present.

- **P mitrale:** this is a broad M-shaped P wave which is a sign of left atrial hypertrophy. It may be accompanied by a sine wave shaped P wave, particularly in leads V1 and V2.
- **P pulmonale**: this is a tall, peaked P wave which is associated with right atrial hypertrophy and right heart strain. It is often seen in patients with chronic airflow limitation and associated right heart failure.

PR interval

The normal PR interval is < 5 mm or 0.20 seconds. It should be measured from the **start** of the P wave to the **start** of the QRS complex (ie it should include all of the P wave). A prolonged PR interval represents a delay in conduction through the AV node. Calcium channel blockers, α-blockers and amiodarone are common causes.

Axis

The axis is estimated by using the vectors of the standard leads I, II and III.

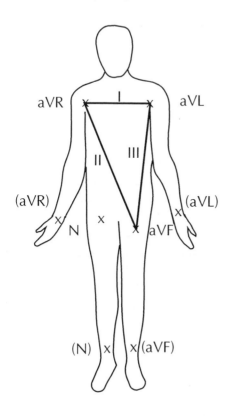

aVR: limb lead attached to the right upper limb

aVL: limb lead attached to the left upper limb

aVF: limb lead attached to the left lower limb

Neutral lead: attached to the right lower limb

fig 1a

Leads I, II and III are 'virtual' leads derived from the vectors of the leads aVR, aVL and aVF. Lead I is made up by the vectors of aVR and aVL, Lead II from aVR and aVF and Lead III from aVL and aVF. Chest leads (V1–6) are shown in Station 1.19.

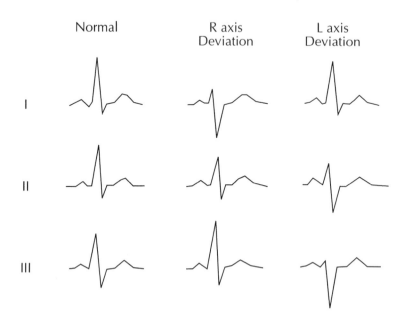

fig 1b: Leads I, II and III showing normal, right and left axis deviation.

There are several ways to 'calculate' the axis. Most experienced physicians are able to state the axis through pattern recognition. Until those heady days, one needs to be able to work it out from first principles. The axis is derived from leads I, II and III. First choose which of the three leads is the most isoelectric, ie when one adds the positive and negative deflections of the QRS complex the sum is nearest to zero. The axis is said to rotate around this lead, which is often lead II. Then work out whether the sum of the positive and negative deflections in the other two leads leaves a net positive or negative deflection for each of the leads. A net positive deflection for lead I moves the axis to the left; likewise a net positive deflection in leads II or III moves the axis to the right. The two patterns of abnormal axis deviation are shown in fig 1B.

QRS complexes

These should be no more than 3 mm or 0.12 seconds wide. Any complexes wider than 0.12 seconds indicate an intraventricular conduction defect or bundle branch block.

To work out right and left bundle branch block (RBBB and LBBB):

RBBB: remembered by **M** a **RR** o **W**

LBBB: remembered by **W** i **LL** i a **M**

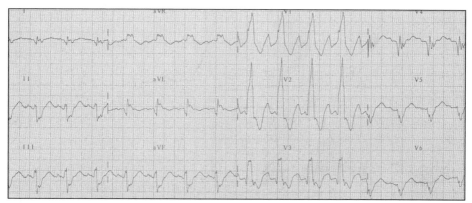

fig 1ci: Right bundle branch block

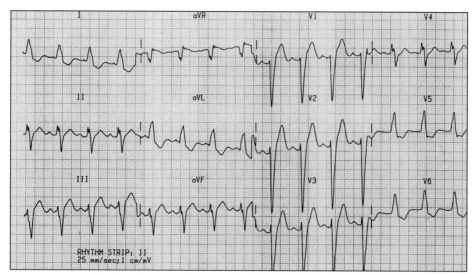

fig 1cii: Left bundle branch block

In practice these simplifications represent:

RBBB: Dominant R wave in V1, and a dominant S wave in V6 and Lead I

LBBB: Dominant S wave in V1, and a dominant R wave in V6 and Lead I

Lead territories

All of the leads, except aVR, represent specific areas of myocardium supplied by the two coronary arteries and their major branches.

II, III and aVF: Inferior leads – right coronary artery lesions or dominant left circumflex

V1 and V2: Anterior leads: left main stem or left anterior descending lesions

V3 and V4: Septal leads: left anterior descending lesions

V5 and V6: Lateral leads: left circumflex lesions

I and aVL: High lateral leads: left circumflex lesions

Signs of ischaemia

Non-critical: ST segment depression T wave inversion

Critical: Q waves, ST segment elevation, T wave inversion

New LBBB

Signs of an acute pulmonary embolism

Sinus tachycardia

Dominant R wave in V1 (represents a right heart strain pattern) right axis deviation

Classically, (although rarely seen) a dominant S wave in lead I and a Q wave and inverted T wave in lead III, termed $S_1Q_3T_3$.

STATION 1.19

Investigation

You are the house officer on call. You have been asked to perform an ECG on a patient complaining of chest pain.

(5 minute station)

1 On the diagram below please indicate the positions of the leads:

  aVR, aVL, aVF

  V1, V2, V3, V4, V5, V6

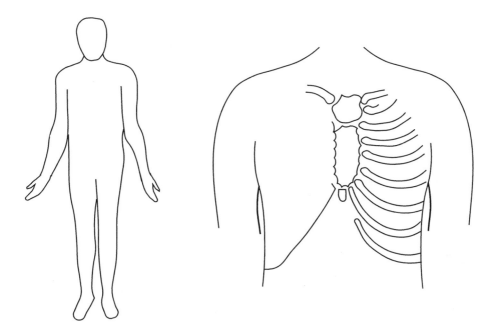

fig 1.19a

2 On performing an ECG on the patient, the trace shown in fig 1.19b was obtained. Please answer the questions below.

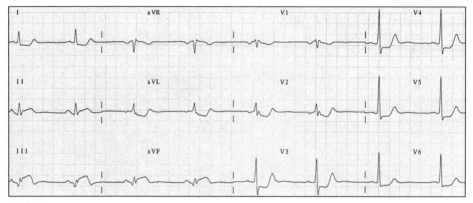

fig 1.19b

(a) What is the rate?

(b) What is the rhythm?

(c) What is the axis?

(d) Is the P wave morphology normal?

(e) Is the PR interval normal?

(f) Are the QRS complexes normal?

(g) What is the major abnormality?

STATION 1.20

Investigation

Please indicate whether the statements below are **True** or **False**.

(5 minute station)

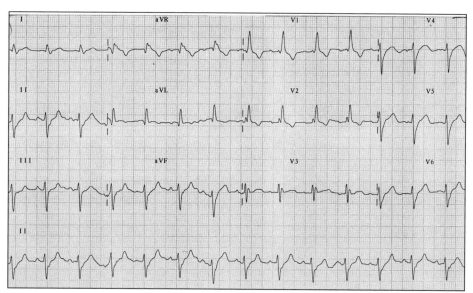

fig 1.20a

1 (fig 1.20a)	True	False
(a) There is first degree heart block	☐	☐
(b) There is left axis deviation	☐	☐
(c) The rate is 66 bpm	☐	☐
(d) There is evidence of left ventricular hypertrophy	☐	☐
(e) There is a left bundle branch block pattern	☐	☐

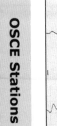

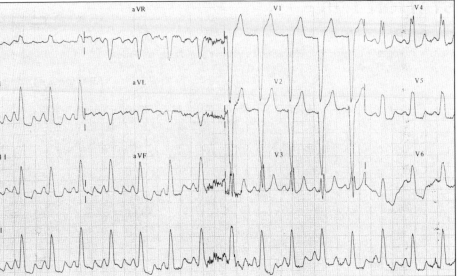

fig 1.20b

2 *(fig 1.20b)*	True	False
(a) There is P pulmonale	☐	☐
(b) There is a normal axis	☐	☐
(c) The rate is 96 bpm	☐	☐
(d) There is a left bundle branch block pattern	☐	☐
(e) The pattern shown is a normal variant seen in healthy people	☐	☐

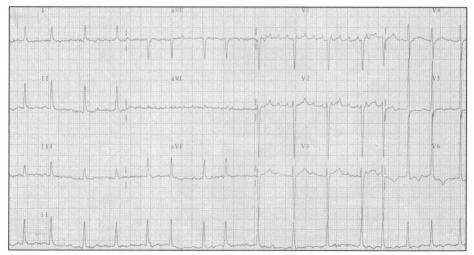

fig 1.20c

3 *(fig 1.20c)*	True	False
(a) There is a normal axis	☐	☐
(b) There is evidence of right ventricular hypertrophy	☐	☐
(c) There is evidence of an old inferior infarct	☐	☐
(d) The patient is at increased risk of stroke	☐	☐
(e) Cardioversion should be attempted if this is a new sustained rhythm	☐	☐

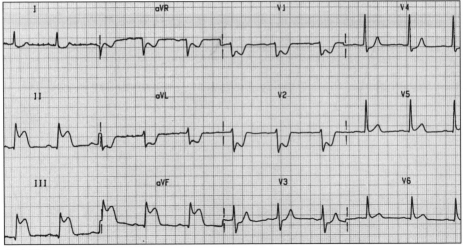

fig 1.20d

4 *(fig 1.20d)*	True	False
(a) The patient is in sinus rhythm	☐	☐
(b) The axis is normal	☐	☐
(c) There is evidence of pericarditis	☐	☐
(d) The patient should be given thrombolytic therapy	☐	☐
(e) This patient is at increased risk of complete heart block	☐	☐

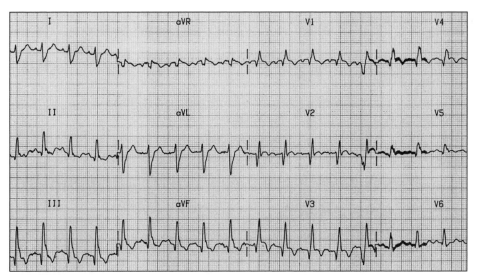

fig 1.20e

5 (fig 1.20e)	True	False
(a) There is a sinus tachycardia	☐	☐
(b) The axis is deviating to the left	☐	☐
(c) There is evidence of an inferior MI	☐	☐
(d) There is a left bundle branch block pattern	☐	☐
(e) This patient will classically demonstrate a respiratory alkalosis	☐	☐

STATION 1.21

Investigation

Please state whether the following statements regarding the radiographs shown below are **True** or **False**.

(5 minute station)

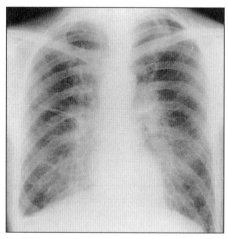

fig 1.21a

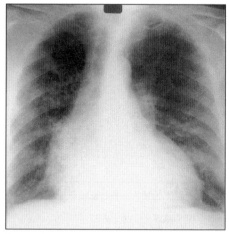

fig 1.21b

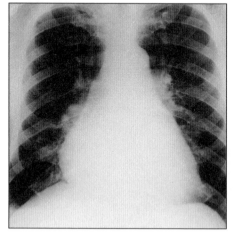

fig 1.21c

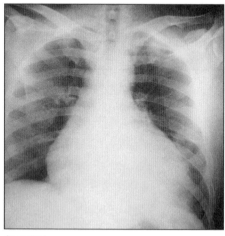

fig 1.21d

1 **(fig 1.21a)**	True	False
(a) This is a poorly centred rotated chest radiograph	☐	☐
(b) There is fluid in the horizontal fissure	☐	☐
(c) The patient is wearing a cardiac monitor	☐	☐
(d) There is blunting of the right costodiaphragmatic angle	☐	☐
(e) This patient should be given intravenous diuretics	☐	☐

2 **(fig 1.21b)**	True	False
(a) This is an AP chest radiograph	☐	☐
(b) There is upper lobe blood diversion	☐	☐
(c) There are Kerley B lines	☐	☐
(d) The cardiothoracic ratio is normal	☐	☐
(e) This patient will characteristically have cannon waves of the JVP	☐	☐

3 **(fig 1.21c)**	True	False
(a) This CXR is overpenetrated	☐	☐
(b) There are hyperexpanded lung fields	☐	☐
(c) There is loss of the atrial appendage	☐	☐
(d) There is cardiomegaly	☐	☐
(e) These radiological findings are associated with mitral stenosis	☐	☐

4 **(fig 1.21d)**	True	False
(a) This is an AP chest radiograph	☐	☐
(b) There is a left pleural effusion	☐	☐
(c) The cardiothoracic ratio is increased	☐	☐
(d) The cardiac silhouette is normal	☐	☐
(e) A cause of this appearance is lead toxicity	☐	☐

STATION 1.22

Investigation

The coronary angiogram shown in fig 1.22b is taken from a 43-year-old man who has recently had an acute myocardial infarction.

(10 minute station)

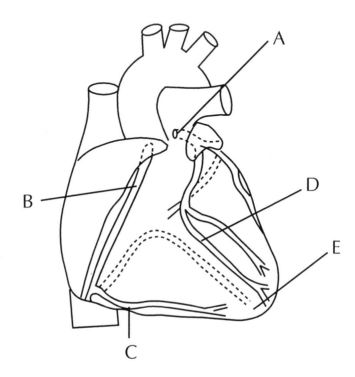

fig 1.22a

Please label the structures (A) to (E) in fig 1.22a and (F) in fig 1.22b: then answer the questions on page 38.

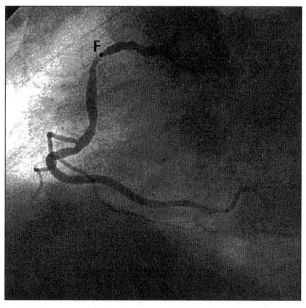

fig 1.22b

1 From the angiogram (fig 1.22b), which ECG leads would demonstrate the infarct?

2 What other changes associated with this type of infarct may be seen on the ECG?

3 What intervention would you recommend for this patient?

STATION 1.23

Investigation

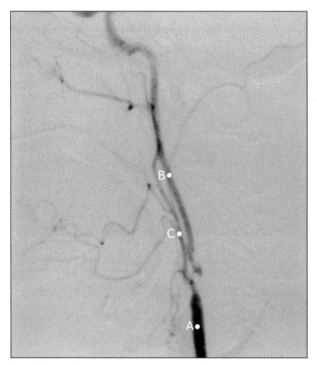

fig 1.23

This is a radiograph of a 61-year-old man with a 6-month history of transient ischaemic attacks.

(5 minute station)

A   1 Name the investigation performed

      2 Name the structures labelled A, B and C

      3 State the abnormality shown

      4 State the principles of treating this condition

B   Answer the following questions by ticking '**Yes**' or '**No**'

1 Amaurosis fugax is caused by:	Yes	No
(a) diminished blood supply to the brain	☐	☐
(b) increased intra-ocular pressure	☐	☐
(c) microemboli to the retinal artery	☐	☐
(d) spasm of the retinal artery	☐	☐

2 A carotid angiogram is commonly performed by accessing through:	Yes	No
(a) the common carotid artery	☐	☐
(b) the brachial artery	☐	☐
(c) the abdominal aorta	☐	☐
(d) the common femoral artery	☐	☐

3 Carotid artery disease is associated with:	Yes	No
(a) Raynaud's phenomenon	☐	☐
(b) diabetes mellitus	☐	☐
(c) hypercholesterolaemia	☐	☐
(d) smoking	☐	☐

4 Carotid artery disease may lead to:	Yes	No
(a) blindness on the affected side	☐	☐
(b) slurring of speech	☐	☐
(c) cerebral atrophy on the affected side	☐	☐
(d) hemiparesis on the affected side	☐	☐

STATION 1.24

Investigation

Fig 1.24 is a radiograph of a 68-year-old man with peripheral vascular disease (PVD).

(5 minute station)

1   (a) What is this investigation called?

    (b) State the abnormality shown

    (c) State two risk factors for this lesion

    (d) List two presenting symptoms in this patient

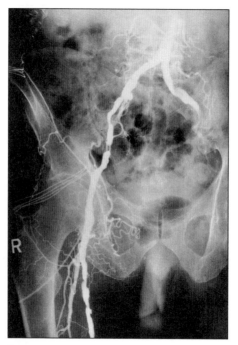

fig 1.24

2 Answer the following questions by ticking the appropriate answer.

	True	False
(a) PVD is rarely associated with smoking	☐	☐
(b) Diabetes mellitus is a risk factor for PVD	☐	☐
(c) Surgery is usually indicated for PVD	☐	☐
(d) Surgical treatment of PVD is usually palliative	☐	☐

STATION 1.25

Therapeutics

You are a house officer on a general medical firm. You have been asked to explain to a 47-year-old woman with newly diagnosed angina how and when to use her GTN spray.

(5 minute station)

STATION 1.26

Therapeutics

1   Please label the diagram of the nephron in fig 1.26 (A) – (K).

(5 minute station)

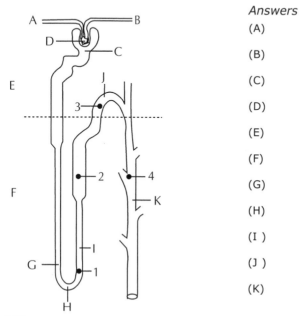

fig 1.26

Answers

(A)

(B)

(C)

(D)

(E)

(F)

(G)

(H)

(I)

(J)

(K)

2   Please indicate at which site, (1) – (4), the following diuretics act:

	Site
(a) Spironolactone	( )
(b) Furosemide	( )
(c) Bendrofluazide	( )
(d) Amiloride	( )
(e) Metolazone	( )
(f) Bumetanide	( )

STATION 1.27

Therapeutics

Please match the patient histories with the most appropriate medication and its described side-effect.

(5 minute station)

Patient history	Drug	Side-effect
1 A 71-year-old man with paroxysmal atrial fibrillation complaining of grey skin, feeling jittery and disliking the hot weather	(A) Atenolol	(a) Xanthopsia
2 A 41-year-old woman with bradycardia and atrial fibrillation on her ECG complaining of nausea and 'yellow vision'	(B) Nifedipine	(b) Peripheral neuropathy
3 A 61-year old man who is 36 hours post acute myocardial infarction now complaining of dyspnoea and worsening wheeze	(C) Sotalol	(c) Fluid retention and vasodilatation
4 A 79-year-old woman with hypertension complaining of flushing, headaches and swollen ankles	(D) Amiodarone	(d) Worsening heart failure and postural hypotension
5 A 27-year-old woman with Wolff–Parkinson–White syndrome complaining of parasthesiae in the fingers	(E) Digoxin	(e) Skin pigmentation and thyrotoxicosis
6 A 51-year-old woman with atrial fibrillation complaining of increasing exertional dyspnoea, and PND, associated with dizziness on standing	(F) Flecainide	(f) Bronchospasm/ asthma

Answers

1 ( ) ( )   4 ( ) ( )

2 ( ) ( )   5 ( ) ( )

3 ( ) ( )   6 ( ) ( )

STATION 1.28

Therapeutics

You are the house officer on call for general medicine. In the hospital in which you work it is policy to obtain verbal consent prior to giving a patient thrombolysis. Please obtain verbal consent from a 46-year-old man who has been 'fast tracked' from the Emergency Department with an acute anterior myocardial infarction.

(5 minute station)

STATION 1.29

Therapeutics

Mrs Debra Thomas is an 88-year-old woman with known myelodysplasia. She has been admitted for a 'top up' transfusion under the Care of the Elderly firm on which you are the house officer. Her last transfusion was two weeks ago and the notes confirm she is blood group A rhesus positive. No abnormal antibodies have been reported. Her Hb, checked yesterday by her GP, was 5.2 g/dl. She is on Flemming ward in St. Peter's Hospital under the care of Dr Little. Her DOB is 13/09/09 and unit number is 123432. She is to have four units of packed cells to start this afternoon.

Please fill in the cross match form (the transfusion form) where details of blood units would be entered by the laboratory personnel and cross-checked by you is shown in fig 1.29a and then write up the blood transfusion on the IV fluid prescription chart provided (fig 1.29b).

(5 minute station)

NEWHAM HEALTHCARE NHS TRUST .... HOSPITAL

REQUEST FOR BLOOD FOR TRANSFUSION AND/OR GROUPING

Patient's surname	first name(s)	sex	date of birth	Ward/dept.	Hospital No.	Ethnic orig.

Consultant.. Signature of doctor
making this request

Patient identified and blood taken by......................... at .... hours on *(date)*......................

Clinical Diagnosis.. Hb ....g/dl.

Nature of operation or other reason for Transfusion ....

Previous Transfusions?.. Group (if known) ....

Reactions?..

Pregnancies?.. E.D.D. ....

Have Antibodies been reported?...

REQUEST FOR:
Please tick or number box as appropriate

Group Only   *Serum will be kept for 7 days*

packs immediately unchecked to save life }

packs urgent   } *Telephone Hospital Blood Bank*

packs whole for use at .... a.m./p.m. on....................................

concentrated cells for use at .... a.m./p.m. on.....................................

For other blood products telephone Hospital Blood Bank

Blood will be issued only if this form is properly completed and is accompanied by a correctly labelled specimen of the patient's blood.

RECORD OF TRANSFUSION Complete in ward. At end of transfusion affix to notes.

PATIENT'S BLOOD GROUP.............. RHESUS (D).......................

The following packs are compatible with patient's serum **ANTIBODIES:**...............................

They will be returned to stock at .... hours on (date) ....

PACK NUMBER	GROUP	RHESUS	EXPIRY DATE	PACK PUT UP BY		COMMENTS	SIGNATURE
				TIME	DATE		

BLOOD TRANSFUSION In the event of a reaction stop transfusion and notify laboratory

Signature...

Date...

F49 NHA809 CSP Ltd.

fig 1.29a – Blood transfusion request form

HEALTH AUTHORITY			24 HOUR INTRAVENOUS FLUID PRESCRIPTION CHART						
DATE			FOR PATIENTS WITH MORE THAN ONE INTRAVENOUS LINE						
CONSULTANT		WARD		Use computer label if available Unit No.					
HOUSE OFFICER		HOSPITAL		Surname				Forenames	
				Address				Sex M/F	
DRUG IDIOSYNCRASY								D of B	
								Weight	

PRESCRIPTION FOR DRUGS TO BE ADDED TO FULL BOTTLE

TYPE OF IV FLUID	VOLUME	INFUSION RATE	TIME STARTED	NURSES SIGNATURE	DRUG ADDED AND SOLVENT	DOSE OF DRUG	H.O's SIG	ADDITION TIME	ADDED BY	PHARM

INTRAVENOUS LINE 1 ; SPECIFY TYPE (eg CVP, Peripheral)   LABEL LINE

INTRAVENOUS LINE 2 ; SPECIFY TYPE (eg CVP, Peripheral)   LABEL LINE

INTRAVENOUS LINE 3 ; SPECIFY TYPE (eg CVP, Peripheral)   LABEL LINE

INTRAVENOUS FLUID THERAPY SHOULD BE REVIEWED EVERY 24 HOURS AND ALL PREVIOUS REGIMENS CANCELLED
NOTE: THE PRESCRIPTIONS FOR INTRAVENOUS FEEDING MUST BE COMPLETED BY NOON TO ALLOW PHARMACY TO PREPARE THE PRODUCT.

fig 1.29b – Intravenous fluid form

STATION 1.30

Therapeutics

You are the house officer on call. You have been called to the ward by the nursing staff to see a patient who has become pyrexial and is having rigors whilst receiving their second unit of a 3-unit blood transfusion. Please explain to the examiner what you would do at the bed side and what instructions you would give the nursing staff.

(5 minute station)

STATION 1.31

Therapeutics: preparatory station

You are the house officer on a medical firm, caring for a 23-year-old woman who has been treated for an OCP induced right lower limb DVT. Please explain warfarin therapy to her.

(5 minute station)

You should mention the following:

1 Adherence: important to take dose prescribed as this will keep patient's blood at the correct dilution; stress importance of not missing doses.

2 Effect: stops blood clotting so easily

3 Side-effects

    a   Haemorrhage: if there are any problems with ongoing bleeding the patient should seek medical attention immediately

    b   Easy bruising

    c   Others – rare: nausea, rashes

4 Warfarin/anticoagulant clinic: visit 1 × fortnight. Warfarin book will explain treatment

5 Duration of therapy: 3–6 months

6 Contraception: must not use OCP; other methods, seek guidance from GP

7 Interactions with other drugs: antiepileptics, antibiotics, you should attempt to answer any questions she may have.

STATION 1.31a

Therapeutics

You are the house officer attached to a general medical firm. You have been asked to explain warfarin treatment to a 23-year-old patient, who was admitted five days ago with a right ileo femoral DVT. She was previously on the OCP. Please discuss the treatment, side-effects and any other relevant information with the patient.

(10 minute station)

Chapter 2:
Respiratory Medicine

Contents

Respiratory History

Respiratory Examination

Arterial Blood Gases

Respiratory Failure

The Normal Chest Radiograph

Chapter 2:

Respiratory Medicine

Respiratory History

Shortness of breath (dyspnoea)

Clarify whether dyspnoea occurs on exertion or at rest. The exercise tolerance should be quantified in terms of:

- Distance patient can walk – on the flat/up a hill/up a flight of stairs
- If immobile – define by activities of daily living (eg washing themselves, dressing, eating, transferring from bed to chair)
- What causes the patient to stop, ie is it shortness of breath; angina; claudication?

The cause of dyspnoea is usually characterised by its associations.

- **Cough**
  Productive or non-productive
  Nocturnal – may be a sign of asthma or aspiration
- **Sputum**
  Colour
  Consistency
  Volume
- **Haemoptysis**
  Volume
  Fresh or altered blood

Haemoptysis is a sinister symptom, particularly in smokers, and should always be taken seriously. Persistent haemoptysis requires investigation.

Causes of haemoptysis

- **Upper respiratory tract**
  Epistaxis; upper respiratory tract infection
- **Pharyngeal lesions**
  Carcinoma
- **Lower respiratory tract**
  Benign and malignant tumours of the lung
  Pneumonia and tuberculosis
  Bronchiectasis
  Abscess

Pulmonary embolism

Trauma

- **General causes**

Blood dyscrasia and coagulopathy

Wheeze

This is a sign of bronchospasm. Causes include asthma, chronic airflow limitation, pulmonary oedema (cardiac asthma) and allergic response.

Orthopnoea

This is defined by the number of pillows that the patient sleeps with. Always ask why the patient sleeps with this number of pillows; not every patient with four pillows is breathless when lying flat!

Chest pain

Principally pleuritic pain, ie sharp pain which is worsened by deep inspiration and is said to catch the patient as they take a breath. Define the pain in terms of character, site, radiation and relieving/exacerbating factors.

Stridor

This is an upper airways symptom of obstruction; it may be caused by lesions or severe infection from the pharynx to the carina of the trachea.

Causes of shortness of breath

- **Respiratory**

Asthma, chronic airways disease, pneumonia, pulmonary embolism, pulmonary fibrosis, lymphangitis carcinomatosis

- **Cardiac**

Silent angina, arrhythmia, pulmonary oedema

- **Neuromuscular**

Guillain-Barré, motor neurone disease, muscular dystrophy

- **Miscellaneous**

Anaemia, obesity, hysteria, ketoacidosis

Respiratory Examination

1 Introduce yourself with name and role; explain the examination and gain verbal consent to proceed.

2 Ensure the patient is correctly exposed and then **Observation**:

Stand at the end of the bed. Comment on:

- The patient's wellbeing, ie well or unwell; distressed or not distressed; shortness of breath at rest.
- **Time the respiratory rate** – commenting on normal, brady or tachypnoea. (The normal respiratory rate is 12 – 15 breaths/minute)

Now comment on the presence or absence of – from the feet up:

- Peripheral oedema and peripheral cyanosis; clubbing of the toe nails
- 'Abdominal breathing'
- Signs of respiratory distress – tracheal tug; use of accessory muscles; intercostal recession; 'abdominal breathing'
- Shape of the chest – pectus excavatum or carinatum and other skeletal deformities
- Neck – lymphadenopathy may be apparent
- Face – central cyanosis; O_2 via mask or nasal cannulae; Cushingoid appearance (from steroids); plethora; pursing of the lips; audible stridor or wheeze.

3 Around the bedside – O_2 cylinder; sputum pot; nebuliser; peak flow meter; temperature chart; O_2 saturation monitor

4 Palpatation

Return to the patient and examine:

Hands
Comment on the presence or absence of:

- Clubbing; tar staining; peripheral cyanosis
- 'CO_2 peripheries' – venodilated; warm; red; bounding pulses
- CO_2 flap – Asterixis (only if clinically appropriate – the coarse metabolic flap is unlikely to be present in a well patient, especially one involved in an examination!)

Face
Reconfirm the presence or absence of anaemia; cyanosis; plethora; cushingoid facies.

Neck

- Feel for lymphadenopathy in all areas – anterior and posterior cervical chain, submandibular, +/- axillae
- Assess and comment on the the position of the trachea

Chest

Re-examine to confirm the presence or absence of scars consistent with:

a Old chest drains – 2nd intercostal spaces (mid-clavicular line) or 5th intercostal spaces, (mid-axillary line (up towards the axillae)

b Aspiration sites – pleural effusions (often posterior or lateral)

c Thoracotomy scars – lobectomy and other thoracic operations

For both the anterior and posterior aspects of the chest you will need to assess:

- Expansion (notoriously poorly performed by undergraduates)
- Percussion
- Tactile vocal fremitus (TVF)
- Auscultation

Make sure you understand how to assess each of these, employing the correct technique and anatomical/ clinical relevance. You may also be asked to demonstrate or questioned regarding vocal fremitus, whispering pectoriloquy and aegophony (all methods of differentiating between consolidation and an effusion).

To complete the examination:

1 Make sure you thank the patient; leave them covered and comfortable.

2 Ask to see: contents of the sputum pot; PEFR measurement; O_2 saturation; temperature recording.

3 As with all examination stations, at the end of the examination you should be able to:

- present your findings in a logical manner
- attempt a reasonable diagnosis
- offer a differential diagnosis of causes
- pre-empt possible questions, eg management and complications.

STATION 2.1   *(Answers – page 207)*

History

You are the house officer on a general medical firm. You have been asked to see a 23-year-old asthmatic man who has presented with acute shortness of breath. He is breathless but able to speak in stilted sentences. His PEFR is 220 l/min.

Please take a history of the presenting complaint with any other relevant history you feel is necessary.

(5 minute station)

STATION 2.2

History

You are a medical student attached to a GP practice. The next patient is a 49-year-old man with a cough.

Please take a history of the presenting complaint and any other relevant history with a view to making a diagnosis.

(5 minute station)

STATION 2.3

History

You are a medical student attached to a respiratory unit. You have been asked to take a history from a 61-year-old new patient in the chest clinic who has been sent by his GP with 'worsening shortness of breath – ?chronic airways disease'.

Please take a history of the presenting complaint and other relevant history with a view to making a diagnosis.

(5 minute station)

OSCE Stations

STATION 2.4

History

You are the house officer on a busy respiratory unit. You have been asked to admit a 63-year-old man from the outpatient clinic with haemoptysis.

Please take a history of the presenting complaint and other relevant history with a view to making a diagnosis.

(5 minute station)

STATION 2.5

History

You are a medical student attached to a GP practice. The next patient is an 18-year-old female A-level student who has come to see the GP with acute shortness of breath and chest pain.

Please take a history of the presenting complaint and any other relevant history, with a view to making a diagnosis.

(5 minute station)

STATION 2.6

History

You are a medical student attached to a GP surgery. The next patient is a 16-year-old schoolboy who is complaining of shortness of breath.

Please take a history of the presenting complaint and any other relevant history, with a view to making a diagnosis.

(5 minute station)

STATION 2.7

Examination

You are a medical student attached to respiratory/ chest firm. You have been asked to perform a FULL respiratory examination on this patient who has:

1 Been complaining of shortness of breath on exertion or wheezing, or

2 Come for his 3/12 outpatient appointment

Please make a full respiratory examination and present your findings at the end of the examination

(10 minute station)

STATION 2.8

Examination

You are a medical student attached to a GP surgery. The next patient has attended complaining of one of the following:

- Mild pleuritic chest pain, or
- Shortness of breath, or
- A dry cough

Please examine the anterior chest – starting at the assessment of the trachea – **you do not need to examine the hands or face**.

(5 minute station)

STATION 2.9

Examination

You are a medical student attached to a GP surgery. The next patient has attended complaining of one of the following:

- Mild pleuritic chest pain, or
- Shortness of breath, or
- A dry cough

Please examine the posterior aspect of the patient's chest and present your findings at the end of your exam. **You do not need to examine the hands or face**.

(5 minute station)

STATION 2.10

Examination

You are a medical student attached to a GP surgery. The practice nurse has asked you to assess the peak flow rate of an asthmatic patient who has recently been treated for a chest infection.

Please assess the patient's peak flow and explain the results to them.

(5 minute station)

STATION 2.11

Investigation

The patients listed below complain of shortness of breath. Please match the patient history with the most appropriate diagnosis and FBC result.

(5 minute station)

Patient history	FBC	Diagnosis
1 A 72-year-old smoker with chronic type II respiratory failure	(A) Hb 12.2 WCC 12.2 Plats 2507	(a) Haemolytic anaemia secondary to sickle cell disease
2 A 61-year-old woman with rheumatoid arthritis on naproxen	(B) Hb 7.2 MCV 104 WCC 4.7 Plats 211 Film – lymphopenia, reticulocytosis	(b) Thrombocytosis
3 A 79-year-old woman with confirmed PE on V/Q scan	(C) Hb 5.4 MCV 65 WCC 6.4 Plats 201	(c) Polycythaemia
4 A 22-year-old woman with mycoplasma pneumonia	(D) Hb 5.4 MCV 102 WCC 12 Plats 173 Film – reticulocytosis, red cell fragmentation	(d) Microcytic anaemia
5 A 27-year-old African man with bony pain and pneumonia	(E) Hb 20.6 Hct 57.2 WCC 20.2 Plats 416	(e) Haemolytic anaemia secondary to atypical pneumonia

Answers

1 ( ) ( )   4 ( ) ( )

2 ( ) ( )   5 ( ) ( )

3 ( ) ( )

STATION 2.12

Investigation

The patients below all have pulmonary lesions on their CXR. Please match the patient histories with the most appropriate biochemical marker and diagnosis.

(5 minute station)

Patient history	Biochemical marker	Diagnosis
1 A 49-year-old man with dyspnoea, wheeze, flushing and diarrhoea	(A) Na$^+$ 145 K$^+$ 2.1	(a) Liver metastases
2 A 56-year-old woman with vomiting and confusion	(B) Albumin 31 AST 57 Alk Phos 567	(b) Ectopic ACTH
3 A 61-year-old man with confusion and seizures	(C) 5-HIAA	(c) Ectopic parathormone
4 A 68-year-old woman with jaundice and 8 cm hepatomegaly	(D) Ca^{++} 4.07	(d) SIADH
5 A 47-year-old man with striae, hypertension, proximal myopathy and oedema	(E) Na$^+$ 106 K$^+$ 3.9	(e) Carcinoid syndrome

Answers

1 ( ) ( )   4 ( ) ( )

2 ( ) ( )   5 ( ) ( )

3 ( ) ( )

STATION 2.13

Investigation
Match the patient histories with the most appropriate diagnosis and immunological marker.

(5 minute station)

Patient history	Immunological marker	Diagnosis
1 A 27-year-old Afrocaribbean woman with shortness of breath and erythema nodosum	(A) anti DS – DNA antibody	(a) Churg-Strauss syndrome
2 A 39-year-old man with shortness of breath, nasal discharge and renal failure	(B) pANCA – anti-myeloperoxidase antibody	(b) Progressive systemic sclerosis
3 A 29-year-old woman with asthma, eosinophilia, purpura and peripheral neuropathy	(C) antiglomerular basement antibody	(c) Rheumatoid arthritis
4 A 67-year-old man with dyspnoea and acute renal failure two weeks after a flu-like illness	(D) antiSCL – 70 antibody	(d) Systemic lupus erythematosus
5 A 43-year-old woman with a symmetrical polyarthropathy and fibrosing alveolitis	(E) cANCA – anti-proteinase 3 antibody	(e) Goodpasture's syndrome
6 A 24-year-old woman with a butterfly rash, pleurisy and bilateral pleural effusions	(F) CD4 helper cell proliferation	(f) Wegener's granulomatosis
7 A 35-year-old woman with Raynaud's syndrome, dysphagia, renal failure and pulmonary fibrosis	(G) IgM directed against IgG	(g) Sarcoidosis

Answers

1 ( ) ( )   5 ( ) ( )

2 ( ) ( )   6 ( ) ( )

3 ( ) ( )   7 ( ) ( )

4 ( ) ( )

Arterial Blood Gases

How to interpret blood gas results

Before attempting to interpret blood gas results it is important to know the normal values and what they tell us.

- **pH 7.35–7.45**; pH < 7.35 – acidosis, pH > 7.45 – alkalosis.
- **$PaCO_2$ 4.6–6.4 kPa**. Think of this as the **RESPIRATORY** component of pH.
- **PaO_2** > 10.6 kPa; If the pO_2 is less than normal, ie hypoxia is present, this implies respiratory failure. To decide whether this is type I or type II failure, one must look at the pCO_2 (see example below).
- **Saturation 96–98%**. You should refer to the O_2 dissociation curve to interpret desaturation.
- **HCO_3^- 22–28 mmol/l**. Think of this as the **METABOLIC** component of pH.
- **Base excess ± 2.0**. This figure gives an indication of the metabolic derangement. It parallels the changes of pH but measures something slightly different. Negative figures imply a net loss of HCO_3^- (ie an acidosis). This negative value indicates the amount of base (ie alkali) necessary to correct the acidic plasma to normal. Likewise a positive value implies an excess of alkali.

The most important elements of the arterial blood gases are summed up below.

Henderson-Hasselbach equation:

$$pH \propto \frac{HCO_3}{PaCO_2} = \frac{\textbf{METABOLIC}}{\textbf{RESPIRATORY}}$$

If the HCO_3^- is raised this causes a metabolic alkalosis. To compensate this would mean one would have to produce a respiratory acidosis, ie one would have to retain CO_2 (slow the respiratory rate significantly) which is impossible acutely. However, in a patient with a chronic respiratory acidosis, ie CO_2 retainers, there may be a compensation by the kidneys with a resultant retention of HCO_3^-. Therefore the pH may be normal. This is termed a compensated respiratory acidosis.

Respiratory Failure

Students often get very confused at the mere mention of respiratory failure. Hopefully this simple explanation will dispel the mysticism on this subject!

By definition if the PaO_2 is subnormal, ie < 10.6 kPa, this implies respiratory failure.

One must then decide whether the respiratory failure is type I or II.

OSCE Stations

Type I respiratory failure

Subjects with a normal respiratory drive use an increase in $PaCO_2$ to increase their respiratory rate, ie hypercapnic drive. Type I failure can be thought of as failure of gaseous exchange, ie anything that may disrupt the passage of oxygen from the alveolar space to the red blood cells.

If they become hypoxic they can be given high flow oxygen, ie 35–100%.

Causes of type I respiratory failure
- Pneumonia – particularly atypical pneumonias
- Asthma
- Pulmonary oedema
- Pulmonary fibrosis
- Pulmonary embolism
- Pulmonary haemorrhage

Remember: all causes of type I failure may cause type II failure when the patient becomes tired or the pathological process in the lungs becomes overwhelming.

Type II respiratory failure

These patients have an abnormal respiratory drive. They are chronic CO_2 retainers and therefore the respiratory centres in the brain stem have converted to hypoxic drive. These patients, if given high flow oxygen, will slow their respiratory rate, eventually leading to apnoea and CO_2 narcosis. Such patients should be given 24–28% O_2, remembering the O_2 content of air is approximately 20%.

Causes of type II respiratory failure
- Chronic airflow limitation (chronic bronchitis and emphysema)
- Obesity (Pickwickian syndrome)
- Chest trauma
- Neuromuscular disease – Guillain–Barré, muscular dystrophy,
- Myasthenia gravis
- Drug overdose – opiates, sedatives

Clinically, patients may be divided into 'pink puffers' and 'blue bloaters'. Pink puffers are thin, pink and classically have type I failure caused by emphysema. Blue bloaters are obese, cyanosed and have type II failure caused by chronic bronchitis. Blue bloaters are the patients who get sleep apnoea (Pickwickian syndrome). Although this division is still applicable clinically, post mortem examination has revealed that many pink puffers have chronic bronchitis and, likewise, many blue bloaters have emphysema.

Consider this example

A 27-year-old man with poorly controlled asthma presents in the Emergency Department with severe dyspnoea. His wife says he has been unwell for three days with a 'cold' and has been coughing up green sputum.

His arterial blood gases, taken on air, are shown below:

pH 7.21

$PaCO_2$ 6.98

PaO_2 7.2

Sats 82%

HCO_3^- 17

Base excess – 5.2

These are the steps you should follow when interpreting any blood gases.

- **Does the patient have respiratory failure?**

The patient has PaO_2 of 7.2 which by definition means he does have respiratory failure.

- **If respiratory failure is present, is it type I or II?**

The $PaCO_2$ is greater than 6.4 therefore this patient is retaining CO_2 and has type II failure. This patient has a low HCO_3^- but if it were raised it would imply chronic CO_2 retention with a compensatory metabolic alkalosis.

- **Is the patient acidotic or alkalotic?**

The pH is below 7.35, therefore there is an acidosis present.

- **Is the pH derangement due to respiratory or metabolic problems?**

The respiratory element, ie the $PaCO_2$, is raised therefore there is a respiratory acidosis. The metabolic element, the HCO_3^-, is low which means there is a metabolic acidosis as well.

This patient has type II respiratory failure with a mixed respiratory and metabolic acidosis. In an asthmatic this is a sinister combination, implying the patient is exhausted and will require assisted ventilation.

Formal respiratory function tests

Early detection and progression of respiratory disease may be followed at the bedside using a peak flow meter. This measures the PEFR (peak expiratory flow rate) and will vary with age, sex and height. Patients with suspected respiratory disease or with dyspnoea of uncertain cause may be sent for formal respiratory function testing. This involves spirometry which measures the FEV1 and FVC and can be used to assess reversibility of their dyspnoea after nebulised respiratory stimulants, such as salbutamol.

The ratio of the FEV1:FVC is normally 75%. A restrictive lung defect causes a reduction in the FEV1 and FVC to a similar extent so that the ratio remains the same or may increase. An obstructive defect causes a relatively larger reduction in the FEV1 compared to the FVC so that the ratio is less than normal.

ie   FEV1:FVC < 75% = obstructive defect

        FEV1:FVC >75% = restrictive defect

The transfer coefficient, TKco, is an indication of how effectively gaseous exchange is occurring. It is therefore affected by the elements that make up alveolar/capillary gaseous exchange:

- The effective alveolar surface – alveolar surface area integrity
- The Hb concentration
- Ventilation/perfusion matching.

Causes of a reduced transfer coefficient include emphysema, fibrotic lung disease and pulmonary oedema. Causes of an increase include asthma, sarcoidosis and pulmonary haemorrhage. The transfer coefficient is useful in distinguishing similar clinical disorders such as asthma and emphysema.

STATION 2.14

Investigation

Match the patient histories with the most appropriate set of blood gas results (taken on air) and the therapy that should be initiated. You should write the inferred diagnoses for each set of blood gas results, eg type II respiratory failure with a metabolic acidosis.

(5 minute station)

Patient history	Blood gases	Therapy
1 A 24-year-old man with a viral respiratory tract infection now presenting with weakness and numbness in the legs and acute breathlessness	(A) pH 7.52 $PaCO_2$ 2.1 PaO_2 14.2 sats 100% HCO_3^- 22	(a) 60% O_2/ heparin
2 A 49-year-old man with acute dyspnoea four hours after being admitted with a large anterior myocardial infarction	(B) pH 7.20 $PaCO_2$ 8.4 PaO_2 4.7 sats 72% HCO_3^- 36	(b) Paper bag/ reassurance
3 A 62-year-old chronic smoker with a cough, green sputum and acute dyspnoea	(C) pH 7.52 $PaCO_2$ 2.4 PaO_2 6.5 sats 86% HCO_3^- 23	(c) IPV/ plasmapheresis
4 A 26-year-old woman with acute dyspnoea, haemoptysis and pleuritic chest pain	(D) pH 7.42 $PaCO_2$ 6.9 PaO_2 8.2 sats 89% HCO_3^- 24	(d) 60% O_2/ diuretics
5 A 14-year-old schoolgirl who became acutely dyspnoeic, dizzy and has carpopedal spasm during a pop concert	(E) pH 7.20 $PaCO_2$ 4.5 PaO_2 7.5 sats 83% HCO_3^- 16	(e) 24% O_2/ nebuliser

Answers   *Inferred diagnoses from ABGs*

1 ( ) ( )   1

2 ( ) ( )   2

3 ( ) ( )   3

4 ( ) ( )   4

5 ( ) ( )   5

STATION 2.15

Investigation

The three patients below have been sent from the chest clinic for investigation of shortness of breath. Their formal respiratory function tests are shown. Please answer the questions below regarding the results.

(5 minute station)

Patient (A)   27-year-old woman with rheumatoid arthritis now presenting with a 6-month history of shortness of breath

FEV1 = 3.0 Oxygen saturation on air – 92%

FVC = 3.8 Transfer coefficient – grossly reduced

Patient (B)   69-year-old man with 2-year history of exertional dyspnoea and an episodic cough.

FEV1 = 2.5 Oxygen saturation on air – 89%

FVC = 3.7 Transfer coefficient – reduced

Patient (C)   22-year-old woman with 2-month history of worsening shortness of breath and fatigue on exertion and repetitive movements.

FEV1 = 3.7 Oxygen saturation on air – 95%

FVC = 6 Transfer coefficient – normal

Which of these patients:	A	B	C
1 Demonstrates a restrictive lung defect?	☐	☐	☐
2 Demonstrates an obstructive lung defect?	☐	☐	☐
3 Has type I respiratory failure?	☐	☐	☐
4 Typically demonstrate type II respiratory failure?	☐	☐	☐
5 Should be treated with nebulisers?	☐	☐	☐
6 Is most likely to have a thymoma?	☐	☐	☐
7 Is most likely to have an associated primary lung cancer?	☐	☐	☐
8 Classically worsen their hypoxia with exertion?	☐	☐	☐
9 May benefit from steroid therapy?	☐	☐	☐
10 May derive benefit from other forms of immunosuppression?	☐	☐	☐

The Normal Chest Radiograph (CXR)

As with all radiological imaging it is important to have a structured approach to the chest radiograph and to know the normal limits. When reading a chest X-ray one must always look at the various components, ie the heart, the lung fields, the hemidiaphragms, the ribs and other bones and the soft tissues. Always check the patient details are correct for your patient before proceeding on to the more technical elements.

PA or AP?

PA (posteroanterior) and AP (anteroposterior) refers to the direction the X-rays travel onto the X-ray plate: a PA plate lies on the anterior chest wall of the patient with the X-rays delivered from behind. AP plates lie behind the patient, with the X-rays directed from the front. The heart appears magnified in AP views as it lies further from a plate lying posteriorly and the X-rays are dispersed over a wider area. Technically, one should not comment on the cardiac size on an AP film.

Rotation

To decide whether a film is centred and not rotated, look at the clavicles and their relationship to one another and the rest of the thorax. On a well-centred film the clavicles are horizontal, directly opposing one another, clearly seen along their entire length, perpendicular to the rest of the thoracic cavity, and equally placed on either side of the vertebral column.

Penetration

This refers to the penetration of the X-rays through the thoracic cavity. Rays that are focused in front of the X-ray plate give poorly penetrated views. The heart and lung markings appear very dense and the vertebrae are not seen. Rays focused too far through the thoracic cavity produce over-penetrated views, with the lung markings and vertebrae becoming very prominent. (Occasionally, over-penetration is used to give lesions in the lung more definition.) .

The heart

The left heart border is made up (from superior to inferior) of the aortic knuckle, the left pulmonary artery, the left atrial appendage and the left ventricle. It is intimately related to the lingual lobe, a part of the upper lobe, of the left lung. Therefore consolidation within the lingual lobe causes the left heart border to become hazy and difficult to define.

The right heart border is made up of the superior vena cava and the right ventricle. It is intimately related to the right middle lobe and consolidation within this lobe causes loss of definition of the right heart border.

The heart size on a PA film should be less than half of the thoracic cavity at its widest point. This is called the cardiothoracic ratio (CTR), and should be < 0.50.

The lungs

The left lung has two lobes, the upper, incorporating the lingual lobe, which lies anteriorly and the lower lobe which lies posteriorly.

The right lung has three, the upper, middle and lower lobes. The right lung is divided by the horizontal fissure, which becomes visible on X-ray when fluid filled.

The lungs are both divided radiologically into three zones. The upper zone incorporates the apices and extends from the apex to the 2nd anterior rib. The midzone extends from the 2nd to 4th anterior ribs, and the lower zones extend from the 4th to the 6th anterior ribs.

Hyperexpansion

To decide whether the lung fields are hyperexpanded, two conditions must apply.

(a) Seven or more **anterior** ribs should be visible, (however this will also apply if a patient takes a deep inspiration). The ribs, in a hyperextended view, often look 'flattened' or very horizontal, as do the hemidiaphragms.

(b) The precise way of establishing hyperexpansion is to draw a line between the costodiaphragmatic angle (A) and the cardiodiaphragmatic angle (B) (fig 2A). A perpendicular is then drawn from the mid point of the diaphragm (x). The distance from the diaphragm to the original line should be 1.0 cm or more. If this distance is less than 1.0 cm the diaphragms are 'flattened' and the lung fields are said to be hyperexpanded.

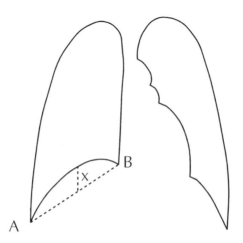

fig 2a

Bones

There should be no more than six anterior ribs seen on a PA film, unless a deep inspiration has been made or there is hyperexpansion. One should comment on whether the ribs and other bones look normal or osteopenic, whether there are any fractures or evidence of arthritis.

The rib spacing is greatly reduced with underlying lung collapse and is termed 'crowding'.

Diaphragm

The right hemidiaphragm should lie 1–2 cm higher than the left. Blunting, or loss of the costodiaphragmatic angles implies an effusion. Always check both costodiaphragmatic angles are present on film. If they are not, one should repeat the film prior to commenting on it. The left hemidiaphragm usually has the gastric bubble below, do not confuse this with pneumoperitoneum caused by perforation of a viscus.

Soft tissues

Always check for calcified masses, air in the soft tissues (surgical emphysema) and, in women, the two breast shadows.

STATION 2.16

Investigation

Please label the chest radiograph (fig 2.16) and answer the questions shown below.

(5 minute station)

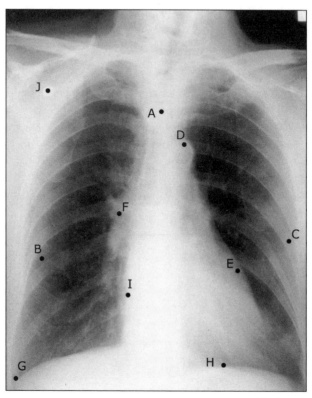

fig 2.16

Answers

(A)   (F)

(B)   (G)

(C)   (H)

(D)   (I)

(E)   (J)

	True	False
1 This is a PA chest radiograph	☐	☐
2 There is evidence of hyperexpansion	☐	☐
3 The cardiothoracic ratio is increased	☐	☐
4 There is calcification in the left pulmonary artery	☐	☐
5 There is upper lobe blood diversion	☐	☐
6 The tracheal position is normal	☐	☐
7 The costodiaphragmatic angles are normal	☐	☐
8 There is a fracture of the posterior part of the left 4th rib	☐	☐
9 There is surgical emphysema	☐	☐
10 This radiograph shows evidence of a perforated viscus	☐	☐

OSCE Stations

STATION 2.17

Investigation

Please indicate whether the statements about the radiographs shown below are **True** or **False**.

(10 minute station)

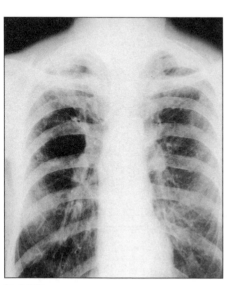

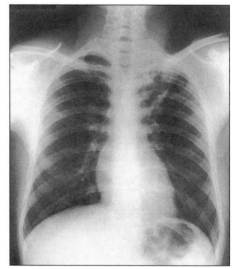

fig 2.17a   fig 2.17b

(a) *(fig 2.17a)*	True	False
1 This is a PA CXR	☐	☐
2 The hilar are enlarged	☐	☐
3 There is pulmonary pruning	☐	☐
4 There is hyperexpansion of the lung	☐	☐
5 This patient has evidence of apical fibrosis	☐	☐

(b) *(fig 2.17b)*	True	False
1 This CXR is poorly penetrated	☐	☐
2 The radiograph is rotated	☐	☐
3 There is cavitation in the left upper lobe	☐	☐
4 One cause of this appearance is tuberculosis	☐	☐
5 The patient requires a bronchoscopy	☐	☐

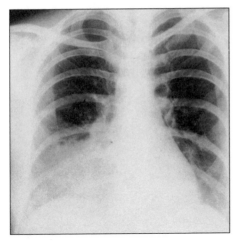

fig 2.17c

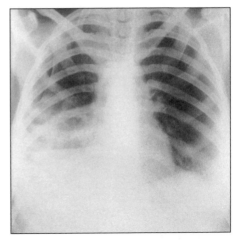

fig 2.17d

(c) *(fig 2.17c)*	True	False
1 This is a well-penetrated CXR	☐	☐
2 There is blunting of the left costodiaphragmatic angle	☐	☐
3 There is evidence of a right lower lobe pneumonia	☐	☐
4 The bones are osteopenic	☐	☐
5 These appearances are characteristic of a Klebsiella pneumonia	☐	☐

(d) *(fig 2.17d)*	True	False
1 This is a well-penetrated CXR	☐	☐
2 The cardiothoracic ratio is normal	☐	☐
3 There is a right sided pneumothorax	☐	☐
4 There is a right sided pleural effusion	☐	☐
5 The lung fields are hyperexpanded	☐	☐

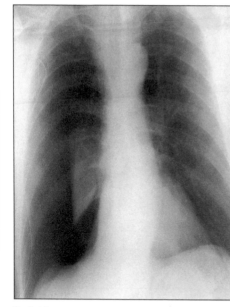

fig 2.17e

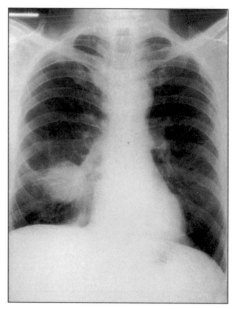

fig 2.17f

(e) *(fig 2.17e)*	True	False
1 This is an AP CXR	☐	☐
2 The costodiaphragmatic angles are clearly seen	☐	☐
3 There is right midzone consolidation	☐	☐
4 There is a chest drain in situ	☐	☐
5 There is evidence of surgical emphysema	☐	☐

(f) *(fig 2.17f)*	True	False
1 This is a well-centred CXR	☐	☐
2 There is a large right apical tumour	☐	☐
3 There is other evidence the patient is a smoker	☐	☐
4 There is tenting of the right hemidiaphragm	☐	☐
5 There is evidence of bone metastases	☐	☐

STATION 2.18

Investigation

Please indicate whether the statements about the radiographs shown below are **True** or **False**.

(10 minute station)

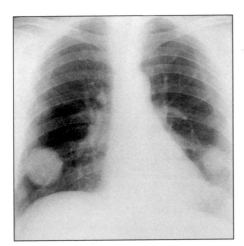

fig 2.18a

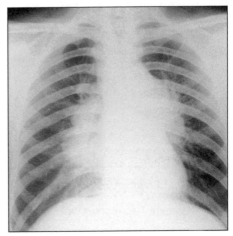

fig 2.18b

(a) *(fig 2.18a)*	True	False
1 This is a well-penetrated CXR	☐	☐
2 There is a left pleural effusion	☐	☐
3 There is tenting of the right hemidiaphragm	☐	☐
4 The multiple pulmonary lesions are consistent with cannonball metastases	☐	☐
5 This appearance is consistent with multiple myeloma	☐	☐

(b) *(fig 2.18b)*	True	False
1 This is a PA CXR	☐	☐
2 It is rotated	☐	☐
3 There is bilateral hilar lymphadenopathy	☐	☐
4 There is evidence of bone metastases	☐	☐
5 This appearance is consistent with sarcoidosis	☐	☐

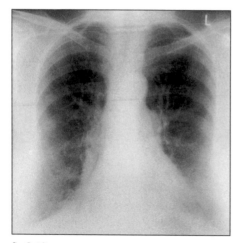

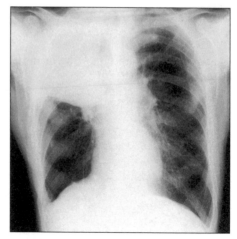

fig 2.18c

fig 2.18d

(c) *(fig 2.18c)*	True	False
1 This is a PA chest X-ray	☐	☐
2 The patient has made a poor inspiratory effort	☐	☐
3 There is evidence of peribronchial thickening	☐	☐
4 There is evidence of cardiac failure	☐	☐
5 These appearances are caused by previous whooping cough infection	☐	☐

(d) *(fig 2.18d)*	True	False
1 The cardiothoracic ratio is increased	☐	☐
2 The left hemidiaphragm is elevated	☐	☐
3 There is evidence of right upper lobe collapse	☐	☐
4 There is right middle lobe consolidation	☐	☐
5 A cause of this appearance is a bronchogenic carcinoma	☐	☐

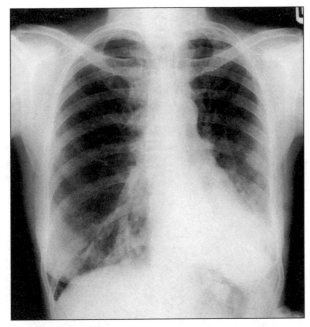

fig 2.18e

(e) *(fig 2.18e)*	True	False
1 This patient has had a right sided mastectomy	☐	☐
2 There is evidence of mediastinal shift	☐	☐
3 There is a left apical pneumothorax	☐	☐
4 There is a 'double' left heart border	☐	☐
5 This appearance is consistent with left lower lobe collapse	☐	☐

STATION 2.19

Investigation
Please label the two CT scans of the thorax taken at the level of the clavicles and the mid thorax.

(10 minute station)

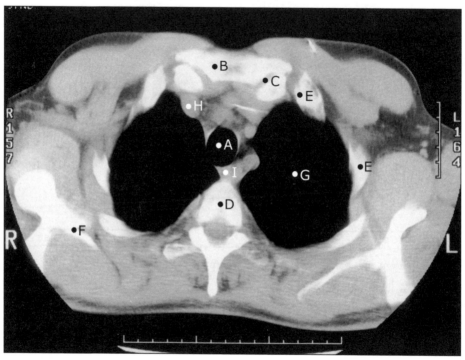

fig 2.19a

(a) Fig 2.19a

Answers

(A)	(F)
(B)	(G)
(C)	(H)
(D)	(I)
(E)	

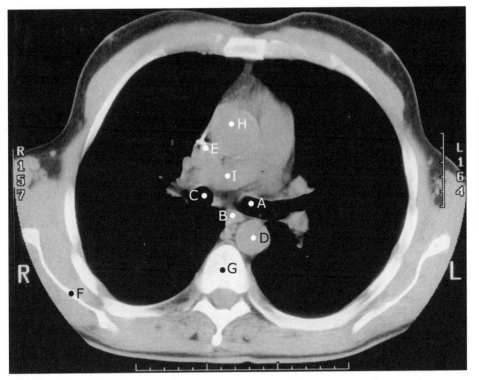

fig 2.19b

(b) Fig 2.19b

Answers

(A)   (F)

(B)   (G)

(C)   (H)

(D)   (I)

(E)

STATION 2.20

Investigation

Please answer the questions about each of the investigations shown.

(5 minute station)

1 A 63-year-old woman presents with central chest pain radiating through to her back.

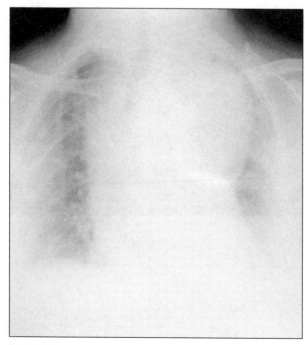

fig 2.20a

(a) What is the investigation?

(b) What does it show?

2 A CT scan of her thorax is then performed

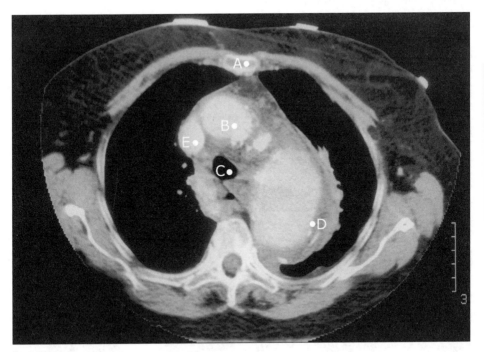

fig 2.20b

Label the structures A–E

(A)   (D)

(B)   (E)

(C)

3 A 27-year-old woman on the OCP is referred to the Emergency Department with pain and swelling in her left leg.

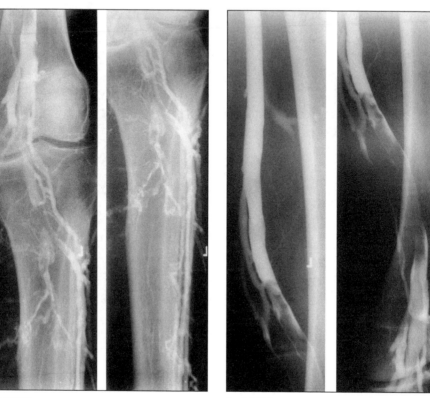

fig 2.20ci   fig 2.20cii

(a) What is this investigation?

(b) What does it show?

(c) What is the further management?

(d) List one alternative mode of investigation for this condition.

STATION 2.21

Investigation

Please answer the questions below regarding the two studies shown.

(5 minute station)

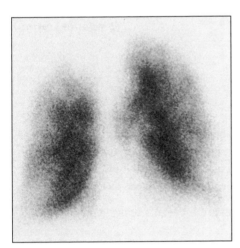

fig 2.21ai

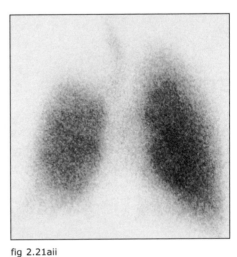

fig 2.21aii

(a)

1 What is this investigation?

2 What do the V and Q scans represent?

3 What do the scans show?

4 What treatment would you recommend?

(b)

1 What is this investigation?

2 What does it show?

3 What do the radio-opaque tubes represent?

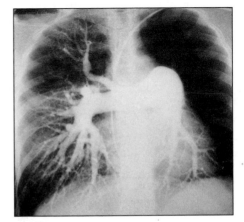

fig 2.21b

STATION 2.22

Therapeutics

You are the house officer attached to the respiratory firm. You have been asked to explain to a newly diagnosed 22-year-old asthmatic how and when to use the inhalers.

(5 minute station)

STATION 2.23

Therapeutics

You are a GP. The next patient is a 31-year-old, poorly controlled asthmatic, who has been placed on long-term steroids by the hospital consultant to improve her control. The patient is very worried about the steroids as she has heard 'they can do terrible things to your body'. Of note, the patient is also an insulin dependent diabetic.

Please explain the steroid therapy to the patient, the benefits and the possible side-effects.

(5 minute station)

STATION 2.24

Therapeutics

You are a house officer attached to a chest unit. The consultant has asked you to talk to a 64-year-old chronic airways patient who is to have home oxygen therapy and does not seem to understand very much about it.

Please explore the patient's understanding and anxieties about the therapy, and explain the benefits to her.

(5 minute station)

STATION 2.25

Informed consent: preparatory
Please read the information below. You have 5 minutes to prepare for the next station.

You are a house officer on a respiratory firm. You have been asked to obtain informed consent from a 53-year-old man who is to have a bronchoscopy and biopsy tomorrow for a large mass in the right midzone on his CXR, which is likely to be malignant. The procedure is performed under local anaesthetic and takes about 20 minutes. The bronchoscope is about as thick as a finger and is inserted down into the 'windpipe'. The instrument is thin enough to allow the patient to breathe.

(5 minute station)

Common complications
- Sore throat postprocedure
- Some chest discomfort
- Drowsiness postprocedure

Uncommon complications
- Bleeding into the lung
- Perforation of the windpipe and smaller airways, causing pneumomediastinum, pneumothorax and surgical emphysema

If the patient incurs a significant pneumothorax or severe surgical emphysema there may be a need for insertion of a chest drain.

If asked directly, you should confirm the mass on the X-ray, may indeed be a cancer.

STATION 2.25a

Informed consent
You have been asked to obtain informed consent from the 53-year-old man who is to have a bronchoscopy and biopsy tomorrow for a large lesion in the right lung, which is likely to be malignant.

Please obtain informed consent from the patient and address any questions he may have.

(5 minute station)

Chapter 3: Rheumatology and Dermatology

Contents

Rheumatology History

Dermatology History

Joint Examination

Examination of the Hands

GALS assessment

Chapter 3:
Rheumatology and Dermatology

Rheumatology History

Arthritis

- Acute arthritis is characterised by erythema, an increase in temperature, swelling and pain of a joint/joints.
- Chronic arthritis is characterised by deformity and pain

Arthritis may also present with acute on chronic disease.

- Age of onset: childhood, adolescent, adult
- Patterns: symmetry versus asymmetry; monoarticular versus polyarthropathy
- Small joint involvement
  Proximal interphalangeal joints
  Rheumatoid arthritis
  Psoriatic arthropathy
  Distal interphalangeal joints
  Osteoarthritis
  Gout
  Psoriasis
- Sacro-ileitis, associated with HLA, B27 diseases – psoriasis, inflammatory bowel disease, ankylosing spondylitis
- Early morning stiffness characteristic of rheumatoid and ankylosing spondylitis

Multisystem disease

Many arthritides are multisystem diseases and one should ask the patient about specific systems involvement. Many of these systemic diseases present with non-specific symptoms, eg malaise, lethargy, fever, myalgia and arthralgia.

- CNS
Aseptic meningitis
Hypopituitarism
Psychiatric symptoms
Cranial nerve palsies (mononeuritis multiplex)
Eyes: keratoconjuctivitis, iritis, uveitis, episcleritis

- PNS: mononeuritis multiplex, peripheral neuropathy, spastic paraparesis
- CVS: myocarditis, pericardial effusion, valvular regurgitation, conduction system fibrosis/ECG abnormalities
- RS: pleural effusions, pleuritic pain, fibrosis, pneumonitis
- GIT: dysmotility and dysphagia; GI bleed secondary to NSAIDs
- Renal: nephrotic syndrome, glomerulonephritis, renal hypertension
- Skin: rashes, eg malar rash of SLE; erythema multiforme; psoriasis
Nail changes: psoriasis; vasculitides
- Raynaud's syndrome: changes of the skin of the digits associated with cold exposure. The digits become painful, cyanosed and then colourless, eventually becoming red.

Activities of daily living

With all arthritides it is important to assess the impact of the arthritis on the patient's everyday functions, particularly mobility, cooking, eating, washing, occupation and handwriting.

Dermatology History

All rashes should be characterised by:

- Site of initial rash
  peripheral or central
  flexor or extensor surfaces
- Sites of spread
  peripheral to central: centripetal
  central to peripheral: centrifugal
- Erythema
- Macular: flattened lesions
- Papular: raised lesions
- Vesicular – vesicles
- Blistering: whether tense or shearing
- Scaling
- Plaques
- Pigmentation and depigmentation

- Involvement of :
  Eyes – conjuctivitis
  Mucous membranes – mouth
  Hair/scalp
  Nails
  Genitalia: urethral and vaginal discharge

All pigmented skin lesions should be defined by:

Size: increasing size or previously unrecognised lesions need investigation

Site: sun exposed areas are common sites of melanomas. The palms and soles do not contain melanocytes and are therefore abnormal sites for pigmented lesions. Other sites where pigmented lesions need to be investigated are under the nails, ie subungal and the retina.

Surface: ulceration/crusting

Shape: change in margins, rapid enlargement is a sinister sign

Satellite lesions: smaller lesions surrounding the original lesion

Similar distant lesions: skin metastases

Bleeding: spontaneous bleeding of a lesion is sinister

Pruritus: itching of a lesion may be associated with malignant change

Pigmentation: change in the colour of a lesion needs investigation

Lymph nodes: associated lymphadenopathy

Metastases: melanomas commonly metastasise to the brain and the liver

Non-pigmented lesions: amelanotic melanomas may be found in nail beds, palms and soles.

Rashes may be manifestations of systemic disease and one should always ask about associated systemic upset.

- Other important factors:
  Drugs/medications
  Allergies – medicines, foods, other environmental factors
  Contacts with similar rash

It is important to take a comprehensive dermatological history, particularly when you do not instantly recognise the rash. If you are able to describe the rash to a dermatologist over the telephone, or a video link, they can often make a diagnosis and give you advice about management.

Joint Examination

Any joint is subject to inflammatory and infective disorders. There is tendency for rheumatoid disease to affect the wrist and hand and osteoarthritis to affect the weight bearing joints or the shoulder and elbow in individuals who have extensively used arm movements in sporting or other activities. A number of congenital deformities occur, severe trauma can damage joints and fracture bones and less commonly, a variety of tumours are encountered. Before examining a joint, it is important to ask the patient about local tenderness and pain on active or passive movement and the usual range of movement. Examination follows the generic headings of look, feel, move (active, passive and walk) and function. Another important component of the examination may include measurement, eg real and apparent leg length in hip disease and is always complemented by radiological investigation.

> **Generic examination of a joint**
> **Look (observe) → Feel (palpate) → Move (passive/active range of movement) → Function (testing of normal functions)**

1 Look/Observation – look for:

- the position of the joint, deformities, swelling, overlying skin changes and muscle wasting.

2 Feel/Palpation – examine for:

- Tenderness, deformities, swelling and joint effusions.

3 Move/Movement – one should assess:

- Active movement (how well the patient can move the joint unassisted) must be assessed first to identify the usual range and any associated pain. Active movement includes weight bearing and walking or using the upper limb particularly to identify pain-provoking manoeuvres. This is then followed by:
- gentle passive movement to identify the full range or flexity of a joint – 'assisted' by the person examining the joint
- the ranges of active and passive movement should then be recorded
- palpate over the joint during movement for crepitus.

Function – assess normal function of limbs and joints.

Measurement identifies muscle wasting comparing two sides if the disease is unilateral, and comparing lengths of normal and abnormal limbs from fixed bony points.

OSCE Stations

Common joints included in OSCEs are:

1 The hip

2 The knee, and less commonly

3 The shoulder

4 The hands are a 'special case' and are commonly included in undergraduate and postgraduate clinical examinations.

5 More recently the GALS screening tool (see GALS – screening examination for the musculoskeletal system. The GALS system Doherty, M et al, Ann Rheum Disease [1993] 51, 1165 – 1169) has also been included as a teaching aid and as an OSCE station. For teaching/learning purposes we shall consider this in a slightly different way – see below.

When examining a joint one should know its normal range of movements.

1 The hip

> Flexion – at least 90 – 100° (limited by the anterior abdominal wall)
> Extension – neutral, ie 0° – 5°
> Abduction – 45°
> Adduction – 30°
> Internal rotation
> External rotation $\Big\}$ in flexion and extension

2 The knee

Flexion – 0 – 135°

Extension – neutral/0°; need to exclude hyperextension

Examination of the knee should include an assessment of the ligamentous stability. Including:

> (a) Anterior and posterior cruciate ligaments – using the 'draw' tests
> (b) Medical and lateral collateral ligaments

Other clinical tests of the knee include:
> (c) Latchman's test
> (d) McMurray's test

3 The shoulder

Flexion – 180°	Extension – 65°
Abduction – 90°	Adduction – 50°
Internal rotation – 90°	External rotation – 60°

Examination of the Hands

When asked to examine a patient's hands one must assume they have reduced movements, pain, stiffness and fixed deformities. So, one must handle the patient's hand as little and as carefully as possible.

Start the examination by sitting the patient comfortably either upright propped up on their pillows or on the bedside or on a chair. Place the patient's hands on a spare pillow palms down. Observe for signs of the common arthritides.

1 Rheumatoid arthritis

(a) Observe for:

Acute changes: hot, painful, swollen joints

Chronic changes: chronic deformity including

- Boutonniere's deformity – flexion (PIP); extension (DIP)
- Swan neck deformity – extension (PIP); flexion (DIP)
- 'Z' thumb
- Subluxation and swelling at MCP joints
- Ulnar deviation of the fingers
- Dorsal wasting, also known as 'guttering' of the back of the hands
- Subluxation and swelling of the wrist
- Palmar erythema; vasculitic nail fold changes

Once you have examined the dorsal surface ask the patient to turn their hands over and lay them back on the pillow. DO NOT turn them over yourself. This is a recipe for disaster and tears for both patient and exam candidate alike!

(b) Palpation

- Palpate for increased temperature and tenderness of the joints
- Gently squeeze interphalangeal joints to assess for synovitis

(c) Function

Ask the patient to complete fine motor tasks such as doing up and undoing buttons and holding a pen or knife and fork. Then ask the patient to demonstrate gross motor skills such as making a fist/testing power of GRIP.

(d) Other tests

Rheumatoid nodules – these classically occur along the ulnar border of forearm. To assess ask the patient to cross their arms over their chest with their forearm exposed to the elbow. Examine for rheumatoid nodules and psoriatic plaques.

OSCE Stations

The differential diagnosis of rheumatoid arthritis is the rheumatoid-like arthritis of psoriatic arthropathy. Differentiating signs include:

- psoriatic nail changes
- psoriatic plaques at the elbow/scalp – hairline

Other common rheumatological problems of the hands:

- Gout – mainly DIP joints/asymmetrical; look for gouty tophi
- Osteoarthritis – also asymmetrical; may occur in the presence of 'burnt out' rheumatoid arthritis.
    - DIP – Heberden's nodes
    - PIP – Bouchard's nodes

GALS Assessment – Gait/Arms/Legs/Spine

This is an extremely useful rheumatological screening tool used in practice. It is very useful for both teaching and learning purposes. We have adapted it slightly as GALS is the way the exam is recorded but perhaps not the easiest way to learn it.

Thus consider the patient in four planes.

Examine/assess the joints and associated structures you are able to see in each plane.

- POSTERIOR
- LATERAL
- ANTERIOR
- ANTERIOR/SUPINE

} Examine/assess the joints and associated structures you are able to see in each plane

OSCE Stations

The examination starts with three screening questions

1. Have you any pain or stiffness in your arms, legs or back?
2. Can you walk up and down stairs without difficulties?
3. Can you dress yourself in everyday clothes without any help?

In the posterior plane, ie from behind the patient – examine

1. Cervical spine – extension; lateral flexion; rotation
2. Normal/abnormal curvatures of thoracic and lateral spine
    (a) Ask the patient to rotate to left and right whilst fixing their pelvis with your hands
    (b) Ask them to try and touch their toes – measure the flexion in the lumbar spine by placing two fingers on adjacent spinous processes and observe the fingers separating
3. Ensure the pelvis is symmetrical/no abnormal rotation
4. Check in the popliteal fossae for cysts (Baker's cyst in rheumatoid)
5. Palpate the Achilles' tendons for tendonitis

In the lateral plane – from the side of the patient

Observe for abnormal curvatures of the spine; abnormal posture and deformities of the hips/knees

In the anterior plane – from the front of the patient

1 Eyes – exclude iritis; keratoconjunctivitis
2 Temporomandibular joints (TMJ) – ask patient to open mouth; move jaw to left and right
3 Cervical spine – flexion
4 Upper limbs
   (a) Shoulders – 'place hands behind head'
   (b) Elbows – pronation/supination
   (c) Hands – test power of grip; make a pair of fists
   (d) Symmetry of the anterior iliac spines (ASIS)
   (e) Deformity of the knees
   (f) Dorsum of the feet/toes

With the patient lying on their back (supine)

1 Assess flexion/extension of the hips
2 Assess flexion/extension of the knees
3 Assess dorsi/plantar flexion of the ankles
4 Assess plantar surface of feet

Complete the examination by formally assessing the patient's gait (this should have been noted as the patient walked into the room!).

STATION 3.1 *(Answers – page 245)*

History

You are a medical student attending a rheumatology outpatient clinic. The next patient is a 23-year-old woman who has been referred by her GP with arthritic pains in her hands.

Please take a history of the presenting complaint and any other relevant history with a view to making diagnosis.

(10 minute station)

STATION 3.2

History

You are a medical student attending a rheumatology outpatient department clinic. The next patient is a 16-year-old schoolboy, who has been referred by his GP with back pain.

Please take a history of the presenting complaint and any other relevant history with a view to making a diagnosis.

(10 minute station)

STATION 3.3

History

You are a medical student attached to a GP practice. The next patient is a 27-year-old woman who has come to see the doctor because of a worsening rash over her cheeks and aching of the joints in her hands.

Please take a history of the presenting complaint, and any other relevant history, with a view to making a diagnosis.

(10 minute station)

STATION 3.4

History

You are a medical student attached to a rheumatology outpatient clinic. The next patient is a 37-year-old woman who has been referred by her GP complaining of painful hands in the cold and increasing difficulties with swallowing.

Please take a history of the presenting complaint and any other relevant history, with a view to making diagnosis.

(10 minute station)

STATION 3.5

History

You are a medical student attached to a rheumatology outpatient clinic. The next patient is a 25-year-old man, who has been referred by his GP with a hot swollen knee and gritty sticky eyes.

Please take a history of the presenting complaint, and any other relevant history, with the aim of making a diagnosis.

(5 minute station)

STATION 3.6

History

You are a GP. The next patient is a 65-year-old woman with headaches and shoulder pains.

Please take a history of the presenting complaint with a view to making a diagnosis.

(10 minute station)

STATION 3.7

Examination

You are a medical student in a rheumatology clinic. The SpR has asked you to examine this patient's hands.

Please make a full assessment including the residual function.

(5 minute station)

STATION 3.8

Examination

You are a medical student attached to a GP practice. The GP has asked you to perform the GALS screening assessment on the next patient who has attended with 'joint pains'.

Please perform the GALS assessment, you will be asked some questions about future management on completion of the examination.

(10 minute station)

STATION 3.9

Investigation

A 24-year-old woman is being treated in the rheumatology outpatient clinic for SLE.

Please study the data shown below and then indicate whether the statements are **True** or **False**.

(5 minute station)

FBC: Hb 9.4 , MCV 102, WCC 6.9, Plat 33, retics 5%

U+Es: Na^+ 139 K^+ 6.8 HCO_3^- 16 Ur 19 Cr 523

Glucose: 4.8

LFTs: Albumin 19, Alk phos 598, AST 135, ALT 213, Bili 34

	True	False
1 The patient has a macrocytic anaemia	☐	☐
2 The anaemia is most likely due to vitamin B12 deficiency	☐	☐
3 There is evidence of haemolysis	☐	☐
4 The patient has a pancytopenia	☐	☐
5 In SLE the thrombocytopenia is usually due to splenomegaly	☐	☐
6 The renal function indicates pre-renal impairment	☐	☐
7 The hyperkalaemia indicates acute chronic renal failure	☐	☐
8 A cause of renal failure in this patient is glomerulonephritis	☐	☐
9 The albumin is consistent with a nephrotic syndrome	☐	☐
10 This patient has a metabolic alkalosis	☐	☐
11 The LFTs indicate a predominantly hepatitic jaundice	☐	☐
12 Gall stones commonly produce the pattern of LFTs shown	☐	☐
13 The LFTs may be deranged due to the drug therapy	☐	☐
14 The haemolysis accounts for some of the hyperbilirubinaemia	☐	☐
15 The patient should have a CT scan of the abdomen as a matter of urgency	☐	☐

OSCE Stations

STATION 3.10

Investigation

Please match the patient histories with the corresponding diagnoses and immune markers.

(5 minute station)

Patient history	Diagnosis	Immune marker
1 A 34-year-old woman with a symmetrical erosive polyarthropathy and subcutaneous nodules	(A) Diffuse cutaneous systemic sclerosis	(a) Anti–Jo
2 A 23-year-old woman with a photosensitive rash and pleurisy	(B) Microscopic polyangiitis	(b) Anti-proteinase 3
3 A 43-year-old man with a cough, haematuria and a nasal discharge	(C) Polymyositis	(c) Anti-DS DNA
4 A 29-year-old man with Raynaud's phenomenon, exertional dyspnoea and renal hypertension	(D) Rheumatoid arthritis	(d) Anti SCL–70
5 A 54-year-old with pain and weakness in pelvic and shoulder girdle muscles	(E) SLE	(e) pANCA
6 A 35-year-old woman with purpura, nephrotic syndrome, pleurisy and haemoptysis	(F) Wegener's granulomatosis	(f) IgM against IgG

OSCE Stations

Answers

1 (   ) (   )

2 (   ) (   )

3 (   ) (   )

4 (   ) (   )

5 (   ) (   )

6 (   ) (   )

STATION 3.11

Investigation

Please match the patient histories with the corresponding diagnosis and HLA association.

(5 minute station)

Patient history	Diagnosis	HLA association
1 A 32-year-old man with uveitis oral and genital ulcers, arthralgia and erythema nodosum	(A) Sjögren's syndrome	(a) HLA DR4
2 A 21-year-old woman with an acute arthritis of the right knee, urethritis and conjunctivitis after an acute diarrhoael illness	(B) Rheumatoid arthritis	(b) HLA B27
3 A 31-year-old woman with a symmetrical polyarthropathy, parotitis, dry eyes and mouth	(C) Limited cutaneous systemic sclerosis	(c) HLA DR3
4 A 45-year-old woman with a symmetrical erosive polyarthropathy, pulmonary fibrosis and mononeuritis multiplex	(D) Beçhet's disease	(d) HLA DR1 [DQ5]
5 A 38-year-old woman with calcinosis, Raynaud's phenomenon, swollen fingers, telangiectasia and dysphagia	(E) Reiter's syndrome	(e) HLA B51

Answers

1 (   ) (   )

2 (   ) (   )

3 (   ) (   )

4 (   ) (   )

5 (   ) (   )

STATION 3.12

Investigation

Please match the patient histories with the joint aspirate results and the correct diagnosis.

(5 minute station)

Patient history	Diagnosis	HLA association
1 A 27-year-old woman with acute arthritis of the right knee severe headache and a purpuric rash	(A) Heavily blood stained fluid	(a) Gout
2 A 51-year-old bank manager with an acutely inflamed interphalangeal joint of the left big toe	(B) Positively birefringent crystals	(b) Spontaneous haemarthrosis
3 A 39-year-old woman with acutely inflamed right knee and intra-articular calcification on the X-ray	(C) Aseptic tap laden with neutrophils	(c) Meningococcal septic arthritis
4 A 12-year-old school boy with factor VIII deficiency and a swollen painful left knee	(D) Gram positive intracellular diplococci	(d) Reiter's syndrome
5 A 31-year-old man with an acute swelling of the left knee, conjunctivitis and penile discharge	(E) Negatively birefringent crystals	(e) Pyrophosphate arthropathy

Answers

1 (   ) (   )

2 (   ) (   )

3 (   ) (   )

4 (   ) (   )

5 (   ) (   )

OSCE Stations

STATION 3.13

Investigation

Please indicate whether the statements about the radiographs shown below are **True** or **False**.

(5 minute station)

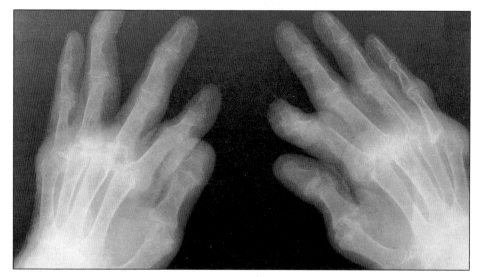

fig 3.13a

1 (fig 3.13a)	True	False
(a) The radiograph shows periarticular erosions	☐	☐
(b) The arthritis is usually asymmetrical	☐	☐
(c) The MCP joints are unaffected	☐	☐
(d) The arthropathy principally affects the DIP joints	☐	☐
(e) These changes may arise in psoriatic arthropathy	☐	☐

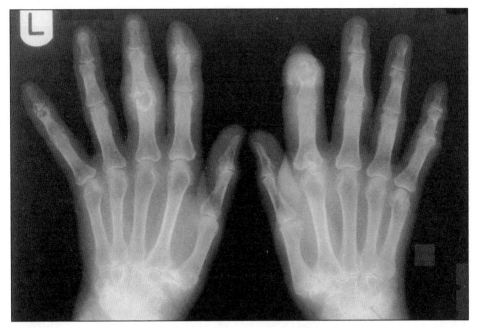

fig 3.13b

2 (fig 3.13b)	True	False
(a) The radiograph shows evidence of periarticular sclerosis	☐	☐
(b) The arthropathy principally affects the DIP joints	☐	☐
(c) This arthropathy is associated with intra-articular calcification	☐	☐
(d) The radiograph shows ulnar deviation of the digits	☐	☐
(e) The changes are consistent with pyrophoshate arthropathy	☐	☐

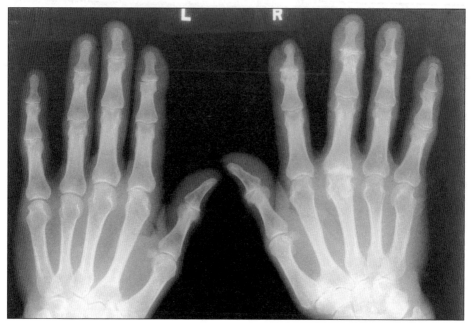

fig 3.13c

3 (fig 3.13c)	True	False
(a) The radiograph shows evidence of osteopenia	☐	☐
(b) The arthropathy shown is associated with periarticular cysts	☐	☐
(c) The arthropathy principally affects the PIP joints	☐	☐
(d) There is an association with HLA B27	☐	☐
(e) The changes are consistent with an erosive arthropathy	☐	☐

STATION 3.14

Investigation

Please indicate whether the statements about each of the radiographs shown below are **TRUE** or **FALSE**.

(5 minute station)

OSCE Stations

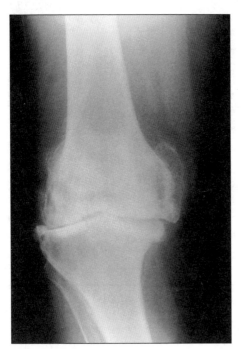

fig 3.14a

1 (fig 3.14a)	True	False
(a) There is relative sparing of the patellofemoral joint	☐	☐
(b) There are several osteophytes	☐	☐
(c) There is evidence of periarticular sclerosis	☐	☐
(d) This disorder should be treated with immunosuppressants	☐	☐
(e) The changes are consistent with a diagnosis of rheumatoid arthritis	☐	☐

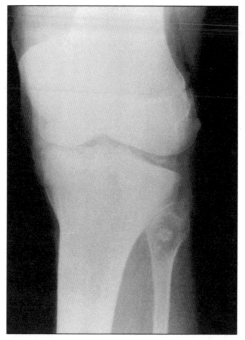

fig 3.14b

2 (fig 3.14b)	True	False
(a) The changes shown are usually symmetrical	☐	☐
(b) The crystals within the joint are positively birefringent under polarised light	☐	☐
(c) There is loss of medial joint space	☐	☐
(d) There is evidence of periarticular cysts	☐	☐
(e) One cause of the intra-articular changes seen is hyperparathyroidism	☐	☐

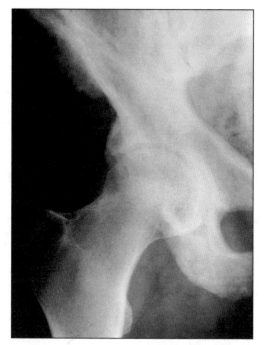

fig 3.14c

3 (fig 3.14b)	True	False
(a) The radiograph shows evidence of cortical thinning and osteopenia	☐	☐
(b) The patient will have a normal serum calcium and phosphate	☐	☐
(c) There is evidence of petrusio acetabulum	☐	☐
(d) The patient has evidence of a pathological fracture	☐	☐
(e) The patient is at increased risk of deafness	☐	☐

STATION 3.15

Investigation

Please indicate whether the statements about the radiographs shown below are **True** or **False**.

(5 minute station)

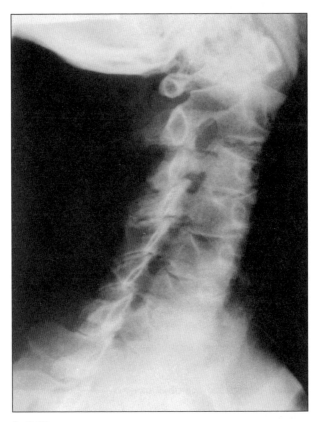

fig 3.15a

1 (fig 3.15a)	True	False
(a) This a lateral radiograph of the cervical spine	☐	☐
(b) All seven cervical vertebrae are shown	☐	☐
(c) There is evidence of osteophyte formation	☐	☐
(d) The radiograph shows disc space narrowing between C6 and C7	☐	☐
(e) There is evidence of cervical osteosclerosis	☐	☐

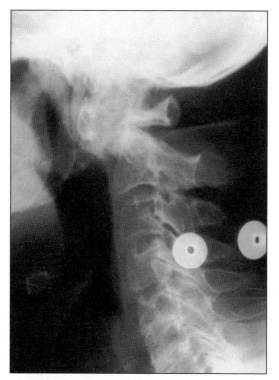

fig 3.15b

2 (fig 3.15b)	True	False
(a) The radiograph shows evidence of soft tissue injury	☐	☐
(b) There is loss of height of C3	☐	☐
(c) The patient is wearing a cervical collar	☐	☐
(d) The condition shown is a recognised complication of rheumatoid arthritis	☐	☐
(e) There is a risk of tetraplegia	☐	☐

OSCE Stations

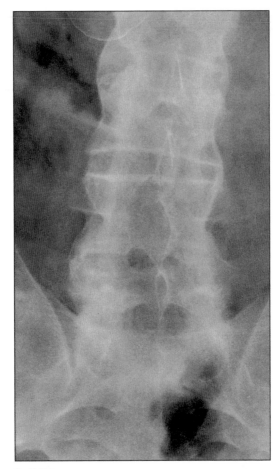

fig 3.15c

3 *(fig 3.15c)*	True	False
(a) The radiograph shows ligamentous ossification	☐	☐
(b) There are syndesmophytes	☐	☐
(c) The radiograph shows evidence of sacroilitis ankylosis	☐	☐
(d) There are osteophytes	☐	☐
(e) This disorder is associated with HLA DR4	☐	☐

STATION 3.16

Investigation

Please answer the questions below regarding each of the investigations.

(5 minute station)

1

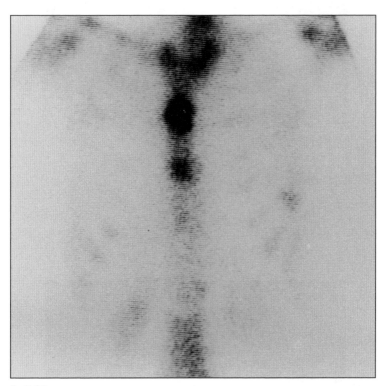

fig 3.16a

(a) What is this investigation?

(b) What is the principal abnormality shown?

(c) What are the treatment options?

2

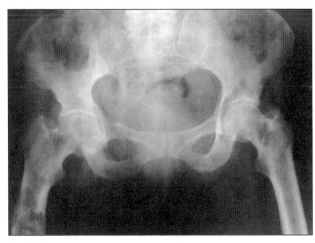

fig 3.16b

(a) What is this investigation?

(b) What abnormality does this show?

(c) List two possible causes.

3

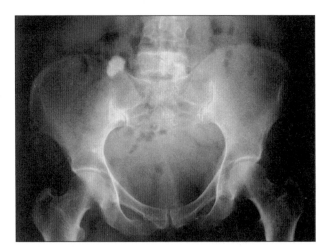

fig 3.16c

(a) What is this investigation?

(b) What abnormalities are shown?

(c) List three common causes.

STATION 3.17

Therapeutics

All of the patients listed below are attending the rheumatology clinic. Please match the patient histories with the drug therapies and most commonly associated complication.

(5 minute station)

Patient history	Complication	Drug therapy
1 A 27-year-old woman with systemic sclerosis now presenting with fatigue and bilateral ptosis	(A) Neutrophilia and thrombocytopenia	(a) Allopurinol
2 A 31-year-old man with rheumatoid arthritis presenting with poor urinary output and peripheral oedema	(B) Corneal opacities	(b) Sulfasalazine
3 A 41-year-old man with severe SLE presenting with acute abdominal pain	(C) Peripheral neuropathy	(c) Methotrexate
4 A 37-year-old woman rheumatoid arthritis presenting with recurrent infections and spontaneous bruising	(D) Myasthenic syndrome	(d) Hydroxychloroquine
5 A 49-year-old man with rheumatoid arthritis and increasing exertional dyspnoea	(E) Nephrotic syndrome	(e) Azothioprine
6 A 61-year-old man with severe gout now presenting with pins and needles in the hands and feet	(F) Acute pancreatitis	(f) Gold
7 A 42-year-old man with primary penicillamine Sjögren's syndrome and worsening visual acuity	(G) Pulmonary fibrosis	(g) D-penicillamine

Answers

1 (   ) (   )

2 (   ) (   )

3 (   ) (   )

4 (   ) (   )

5 (   ) (   )

6 (   ) (   )

7 (   ) (   )

STATION 3.18

History

You are a medical student attached to a dermatology clinic. The next patient is a 36-year-old woman who presents with the rash shown in fig 3.18. Please take a history of the presenting complaint with a view to making a diagnosis.

(10 minute station)

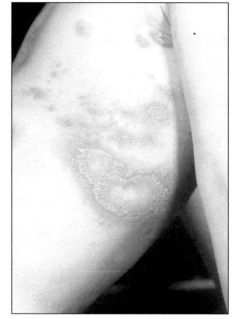

fig 3.18

STATION 3.19

History

You are a GP new to this practice. The next patient is a 24-year-old woman with a fair complexion and multiple 'freckles'. She would like you to look at one of the freckles on her thigh shown in fig 3.19, which has become unsightly. Please take a history to assess this lesion with a view to referring her to a dermatologist.

(10 minute station)

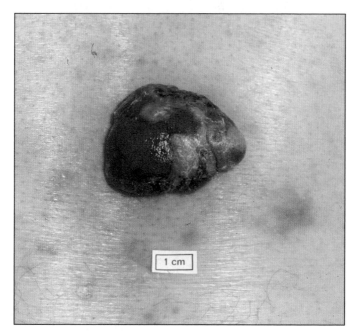

1 cm

fig 3.19

STATION 3.20

Examination

The patients shown in figs 3.20a–d all have nail disorders. Please indicate whether the statements regarding each picture are **True** or **False**.

(5 minute station)

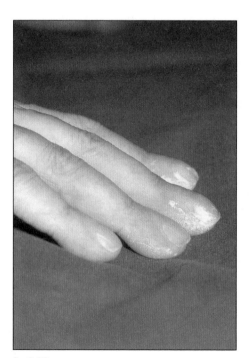

fig 3.20a

1 (fig 3.20a)	True	False
(a) The nail has an increased angle	☐	☐
(b) The nail bed will be 'boggy'	☐	☐
(c) This disorder may be congenital	☐	☐
(d) A recognised cause is coeliac disease	☐	☐
(e) This disorder is associated with acromegaly	☐	☐

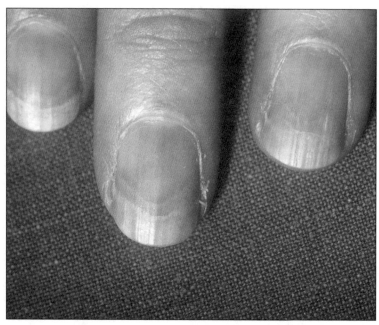

fig 3.20b

2 (fig 3.20b)	True	False
(a) This patient shows longitudinal ridging of the nail	☐	☐
(b) This disorder is associated with squamous cell carcinoma of the lung	☐	☐
(c) The nail bed is normal	☐	☐
(d) This disorder is associated with HLA B27	☐	☐
(e) This disorder is associated with thyroid disease	☐	☐

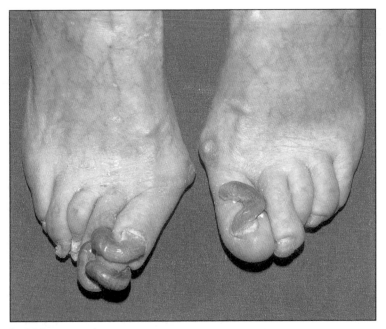

fig 3.20c

3 (fig 3.20c)	True	False
(a) This disorder is caused by a bacterial infection	☐	☐
(b) There is evidence of nail bed onychogryphosis	☐	☐
(c) This is an autoimmune disorder	☐	☐
(d) The disorder shown is associated with carcinoma of the stomach	☐	☐
(e) The disorder shown is benign	☐	☐

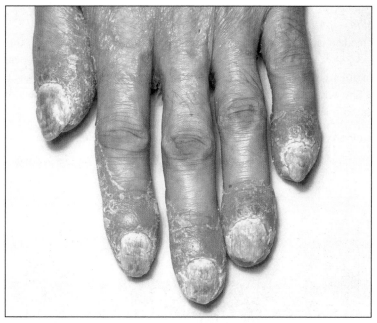

fig 3.20d

4 (fig 3.20d)	True	False
(a) The nail shows evidence of pitting and ridging	☐	☐
(b) The nail bed is fluctuant	☐	☐
(c) The patient may have subcutaneous nodules	☐	☐
(d) The patient may have plaques over the flexor surfaces of their elbows	☐	☐
(e) This patient has increased chance of being HLA B27 positive	☐	☐

STATION 3.21

Examination – pigmented lesion of the right lower limb

You are a medical student and have been asked to examine this lesion on the right leg (figure 3.21) of a 33-year-old lady. She has noticed it to be enlarging over the last nine months but denies there has been any discomfort, discharge, bleeding or ulceration. She has otherwise been well. She has two children, is on a low oestrogen pill and has no relevant past family history.

Please examine and describe the lesion and any other associated findings.

(5 minute station)

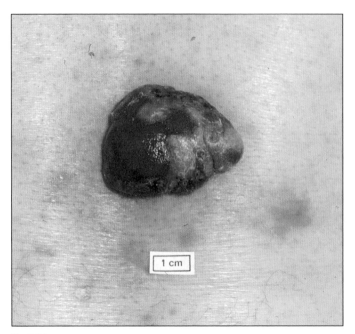

fig 3.21

Chapter 4:
Orthopaedics and Trauma

Contents

Care and Assessment of the injured patient

Chapter 4:

Orthopaedics and Trauma
Care and Assessment of the Injured Patient

The care of the injured patient begins in an emergency setting and the immediate response of the trauma team is directed towards keeping the patient alive, preventing exacerbation of his injuries and deterioration of his vital functions. This involves maintenance of the airway and respiration, cervical spine stabilisation, controlling external haemorrhage and supporting the circulation by obtaining vascular access. Pain relief is administered when the initial survey is completed and the general state stabilised.

Head injuries call for the immediate assessment and monitoring of cerebral function; they are diagnosed by neurological signs that localise the intracranial injury and confirmed by a CT head scan. Cervical spinal injury must be suspected in the unconscious patient and in those with head or thoracic injuries. Displaced limb fractures are gently realigned to alleviate pain and reduce haemorrhage.

Soft tissue injuries are explored and debrided and usually closed secondarily. Visceral injuries must be recognised early as they are usually life-threatening. Thoracic injuries call for ventilatory and circulatory support to ensure adequate lung perfusion and gaseous exchange. Abdominal injuries may result in peritoneal contamination and/or haemorrhage and call for urgent surgical assessment.

The management of a burn injury begins with a brief history of the accident and assessment of the extent and severity of the injury. An inhalation injury requires careful monitoring of respiratory function for signs of deterioration. The local treatment of a burn wound is debridement or excision with overgrafting. Fluid loss from the burn surface is calculated according to burn formulae and replaced. Adequate parenteral analgesia must be administered early. Prophylactic antibiotics are indicated. The emotional impact of a burn injury on the patient, relatives and carers is more evident than in other types of injury and psychological support and counselling must be given.

A survey of injuries to the various anatomic regions may be as follows:

Head
Document the level of consciousness and search for scalp lacerations or bruising that may indicate an underlying fracture. A CT scan is indicated for patients with a GCS score of 12 or less on admission.

If the patient is comatose or is rapidly losing consciousness, suspect a diffuse or focal brain injury. Intracranial bleeding from contusions or lacerations must be diagnosed early as emergency decompression is life-saving and limits the neurological sequelae of cerebral compression. It is essential patients are monitored neurologically with specific emphasis on pupil size.

Face

- Check airway patency and breathing. Examine the eyes before periorbital swelling closes the eyelids.
- Palpate for obvious maxillary or mandibular fractures. Obtain a radiograph of the facial bones.

Spine

Cervical or upper thoracic spinal injury is suspected if there is unconsciousness; flaccid areflexia (flaccid anal sphincter tone or loss of bladder control); diaphragmatic breathing; ability to flex but not extend the elbow; loss of sensation below the injury; hypotension with bradycardia (in the absence of haemorrhage) and priapism (an uncommon but characteristic sign). Obtain a lateral cervical spine radiograph showing C7 and T1 vertebrae.

Chest

The signs of a tension pneumo- or haemothorax are:

- skin bruising, cyanosis and respiratory distress
- paradoxical movements in a flail chest
- tracheal shift to the opposite side
- absent or reduced breath sounds at site of injury and soft tissue crepitus.
- Obtain anteroposterior and lateral chest radiographs.

Abdomen

The signs are seat belt skin bruising; rigid or tender abdomen with rebound and absent bowel sounds. Abdominal distension with hypotension suggests visceral injury and/or haemorrhage. Obtain a diagnostic peritoneal lavage or an ultrasound scan; the latter should only be performed on a stable patient. A pelvic ring fracture or disruption is often associated with abdominal or pelvic visceral injuries and produces significant internal haemorrhage.

Limbs

Limb fractures and joint injuries are often missed in patients with multiple or severe trauma. Long bone fractures are usually obvious from the history and local signs. Feel for pulses and other signs of ischaemia distal to the fracture to ensure integrity of blood flow. Exclude compartment syndrome by ascertaining sensation and perfusion distally. Obtain radiographs of the injured limb in two planes to include the joints above and below the fracture.

STATION 4.1 *(Answers – page 275)*

History

You are a medical student attending an orthopaedic clinic. The next patient is a 43-year-old hospital porter complaining of chronic backache.

Please take a history of the presenting complaint and any other relevant history, with a view to making a diagnosis.

(5 minute station)

STATION 4.2

History

You are a medical student in an orthopaedic clinic. The next patient complains of a wry neck with pain and stiffness.

Please take a history of her presenting complaint, and any other relevant history, with a view to making a diagnosis.

(5 minute station)

STATION 4.3

Examination

You are a medical student attached to an orthopaedic firm. You are asked to examine the cervical spine of the next patient who sustained a whip lash injury three weeks previously and is wearing a collar.

(5 minute station)

STATION 4.4

Examination

You are a medical student attached to an orthopaedic firm. The next patient has been referred by his GP for 'right knee problems'. Please examine his knees with a view to making a diagnosis.

(5 minute station)

STATION 4.5

Examination

You are a medical student attending the orthopaedic clinic. You are asked to examine the hip joint of a 69-year-old man who complains of pain and stiffness in his right hip when walking short distances.

(10 minute station)

STATION 4.6

Examination

You are a medical student attached to an orthopaedic clinic. You have been asked by the SpR to examine the shoulder of the next patient who is a 43-year-old woman, complaining of pain and stiffness when raising the arm above the horizontal plane.

(5 minute station)

OSCE Stations

STATION 4.7

Examination

Fig 4.7 demonstrates a left wrist fracture. What type of fracture is this? Please demonstrate the closed reduction of the fracture in the subject (manikin) and how you would apply local anaesthetic prior to reduction.

(5 minute station)

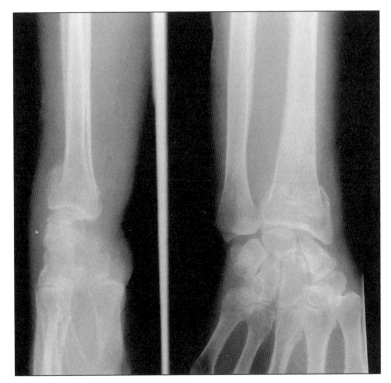

fig 4.7

STATION 4.8

Examination

An adult who sustained a closed head injury is depicted by a manikin.

(5 minute station)

1 Please demonstrate how you would assess the level of consciousness.

2 Please demonstrate three clinical tests to detect cerebral compression/injury.

STATION 4.9

Examination

A ship's gangway, 16 feet above ground level, collapsed during boarding, injuring four ferry passengers who were on it. Clinical observations in the primary survey are as follows:

(5 minute station)

	Patient A	Patient B	Patient C	Patient D
Age and sex	46-year-old Male	34-year-old Female	29-year-old Female	52-year-old Male
Pulse rate	140	120	100	150
Respiratory rate	40	32	20	40
Systolic blood pressure	65	140	120	80
GCS	8	11	14	12

1 Please calculate the Revised Trauma Score (RTS) for each patient from the scoring system given below.

2 How would you prioritise these patients for treatment? Please discuss your reasons.

Revised trauma scoring	Score allocated	
A Respiratory rate	10–24	4
	24–35	3
	> 35	2
	1–9	1
B Systolic blood pressure	> 89	4
	70–89	3
	50–69	2
	1–49	1
C GCS	13–15	4
	9–12	3
	6–8	2
	4–5	1

Revised Trauma Score A + B + C

STATION 4.10

Examination

This 36-year-old woman pedestrian was run over by a motor vehicle. She complained of severe pain in her back and side and was found to have frank haematuria.

(5 minute station)

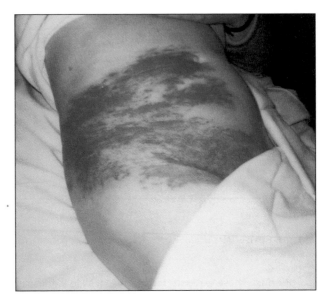

fig 4.10

1 Please describe the features observed in fig 4.10.

2 State the mechanism of the injury.

3 State the likely cause of the haematuria and list two imaging procedures that may demonstrate the injury sustained.

4 List three other structures that are susceptible to injury in this accident.

STATION 4.11

Examination

To attempt this station someone should act as the injured party. All the equipment needed can be found in the Emergency Department.

You are a medical student in the Emergency Department, when a 20-year-old woman is admitted with a suspected cervical fracture sustained in a trampolining accident. Her airway is clear, and she is breathing normally.

(5 minute station)

1 What equipment is required for emergency neck stabilisation?

2 Please stabilise the patient's neck with the equipment described.

3 Assess the integrity of the cervical spine and cord.

STATION 4.12

Examination

A patient (represented by a manikin) is brought to the Emergency Department with a closed fracture of the left femur.

(5 minute station)

1 Please carry out a clinical survey of the injured limb, stating your objectives.

Please answer the following questions by ticking the appropriate column

	True	False
2 A poor pulse distal to a limb fracture should be assumed to be due to vascular injury and not spasm	☐	☐
3 Diagnostic clinical signs of a limb fracture are:		
(a) Deformity	☐	☐
(b) Swelling	☐	☐
(c) Crepitus	☐	☐
(d) Abnormal movement	☐	☐

OSCE Stations

	True	False
4 Compartment syndrome in a limb may be caused by:		
(a) A fracture	☐	☐
(b) A nerve injury	☐	☐
(c) A cold injury	☐	☐
(d) A crush injury	☐	☐
(e) A burn injury	☐	☐
(f) Revascularisation of an ischaemic limb	☐	☐

STATION 4.13

Investigation

(5 minute station)

This is a post-operative radiograph of a limb injury.

1 Name the bones involved and the components used in the treatment.

2 Name the technique used.

3 Which of the following conditions are appropriately treated
with this technique?

(Please tick the appropriate column.)

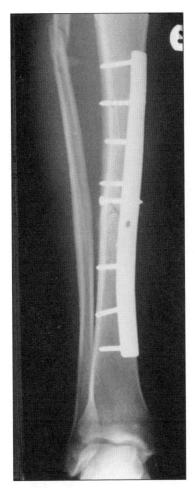

fig 4.13

(fig 4.13)	True	False
(a) Fractures that are unstable and are prone to displacement following reduction	☐	☐
(b) Fractures that cannot be reduced without operation	☐	☐
(c) Fractures that unite poorly or slowly	☐	☐
(d) Multiple fractures that require early and definitive treatment to reduce the risk of general complications	☐	☐
(e) Compound fractures	☐	☐

STATION 4.14

Investigation

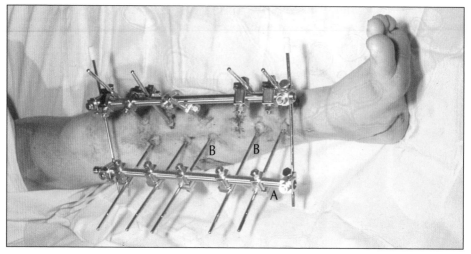

fig 4.14

Fig 4.14 shows a fracture that has been treated surgically.

(5 minute station)

1 Name the bone(s) involved and the components A and B used in the treatment.

2 Name the technique used.

3 Answer the following questions on this technique by ticking the appropriate column.

	True	False
(a) The patient should be encouraged to weight bear on that limb immediately following reduction	☐	☐
(b) This method is suitable for infected or contaminated fractures	☐	☐
(c) This method is suitable for fractures in children	☐	☐
(d) A common complication of this method is delayed healing due to over-distraction	☐	☐
(e) This method is suitable for compound fractures	☐	☐

STATION 4.15

Investigation

Figs 4.15a–c are chest, pelvic and abdominal radiographs of two adults injured in a road traffic accident.

(5 minute station)

1 Please list two positive findings in fig 4.15a.

2 State a positive finding in fig 4.15b and in fig 4.15c.

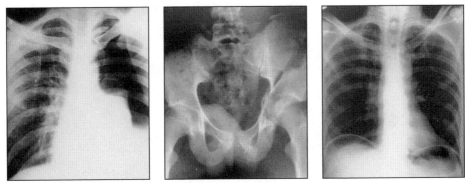

fig 4.15a   fig 4.15b   fig 4.15c

3 Indicate how you would conduct a primary survey of their injuries by ticking the appropriate columns in response to the following statements.

	True	False
(a) Immediately allocate the patients to major, intermediate and minor injury categories	☐	☐
(b) Ascertain whether they are able to walk	☐	☐
(c) Assess their neurological status	☐	☐
(d) Assess their breathing and ventilation	☐	☐
(e) Ascertain the mechanism of their injuries	☐	☐
(f) Completely undress the patient	☐	☐
(g) Protect patients from hypothermia	☐	☐
(h) Take a brief history of events leading to the accident	☐	☐

STATION 4.16

Investigation

This is a radiograph of a 16-year-old girl who presented with a spinal deformity.

(5 minute station)

1

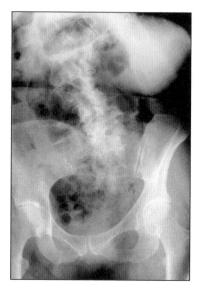

fig 4.16

(a) What is the abnormality seen?

(b) How would you measure the spinal deformity?

(c) Please comment on the aetiology of this condition.

(d) State the principles of treating this condition.

2 Please answer the following questions by ticking the appropriate column.

	True	False
(a) Spinal bracing usually corrects this deformity before adulthood	☐	☐
(b) Surgical correction is feasible at any age	☐	☐
(c) Spinal cord lesions are common in this condition	☐	☐
(d) Muscle palsy is the usual cause of this condition in children and adolescents	☐	☐

STATION 4.17

Investigation

The CT head scans shown below are taken from patients who have incurred a head injury.

Please indicate whether the statements below are **True** or **False**.

(5 minute station)

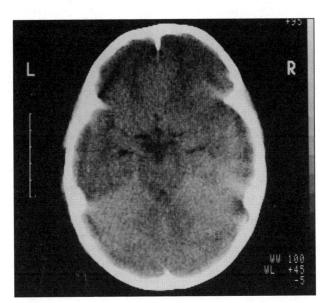

fig 4.17a

1 (fig 4.17a)	True	False
(a) This is a CT head scan with contrast	☐	☐
(b) There is evidence of midline shift	☐	☐
(c) There is evidence of hydrocephalus	☐	☐
(d) There is evidence of cerebral oedema	☐	☐
(e) The patient would benefit from a mannitol infusion	☐	☐

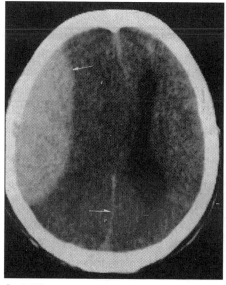

fig 4.17b

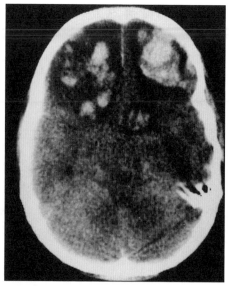

fig 4.17c

2 (fig 4.17b)	True	False
(a) There is evidence of an occipital fracture	☐	☐
(b) There is subdural haemorrhage	☐	☐
(c) This injury can be produced by a punch in a boxing match	☐	☐
(d) The condition shown classically produces a 'period of lucidity' prior to loss of consciousness	☐	☐
(e) The patient would benefit from immediate neurosurgical intervention	☐	☐

3 (fig 4.17c)	True	False
(a) This is a CT head scan with contrast	☐	☐
(b) There is evidence of midline shift	☐	☐
(c) The patient would benefit from nimodipine	☐	☐
(d) The prognosis is independent of the GCS score on admission	☐	☐
(e) There is evidence of intracerebral bleeding	☐	☐

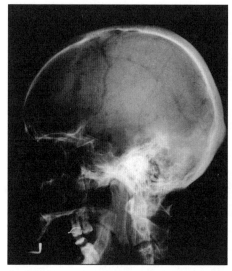

fig 4.17d

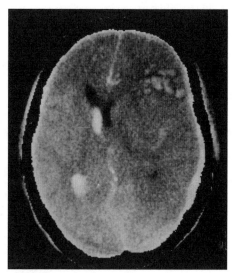

fig 4.17e

4 (fig 4.17d)	**True**	**False**
(a) This is an AP skull X-ray	☐	☐
(b) There is a frontoparietal fracture	☐	☐
(c) This injury may produce a CSF leak	☐	☐
(d) MRI rather than CT is a better modality to image this condition	☐	☐
(e) This injury is likely to have been incurred through a knife wound	☐	☐

5 (fig 4.17e)	**True**	**False**
(a) There is evidence of hydrocephalus	☐	☐
(b) There is midline shift towards the right	☐	☐
(c) There is evidence of intracerebral blood	☐	☐
(d) This condition is often associated with cerebral oedema	☐	☐
(e) This patient should have immediate neurosurgical intervention	☐	☐

STATION 4.18

Treatment
A model of an upper limb depicts a recently sustained 'clean', soft tissue wound.

(10 minute station)

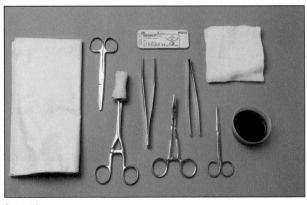

fig 4.18

1 Demonstrate, using the 'minor ops' set provided (fig 4.18), how you would treat the wound in a living subject.

2 The following factors increase the incidence of wound infection.

Answer by ticking the appropriate column.

	True	False
(a) Wounds over one hour old at presentation	☐	☐
(b) Crush injury to surrounding tissue	☐	☐
(c) Presence of shattered glass particles	☐	☐
(d) Use of 2% lidocaine as a local anaesthetic	☐	☐
(e) Use of 1% lidocaine with adrenaline as a local anaesthetic	☐	☐
(f) Loosely tied skin sutures	☐	☐
(g) High wound vascularity	☐	☐
(h) Inadequate haemostasis	☐	☐
(i) Chronic use of steroids	☐	☐
(j) High impact causative force	☐	☐

STATION 4.19

Treatment

An adult, 'depicted by a manikin', has sustained a right sided traumatic tension pneumothorax.

(5 minute station)

1 Please demonstrate the steps you would take in treating this condition, using the equipment on the sterile 'set' provided (fig 4.19a).

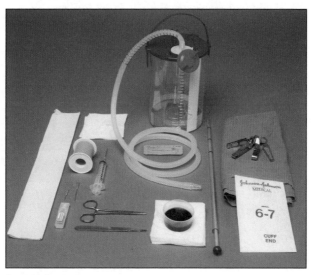

fig 4.19a

(a) Skin prep solution, sterile drapes and dressings

(b) 1% lidocaine in two ampoules, with syringe and needle

(c) Scalpel and non-absorbable suture material

(d) Chest drain with introducer and artery forceps

(e) Water-seal bottle and connecting tubing

2 Fig 4.19b is a radiograph of a patient with a tension pneumothorax. Identify the lesions labelled A, B and C.

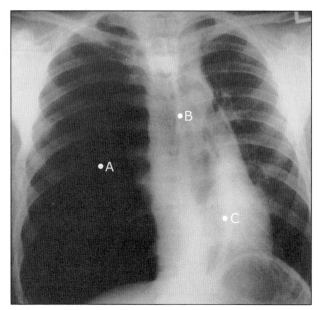

fig 4.19b

Answers

(A)   (C)   (B)

STATION 4.20

Treatment

Fig 4.20 shows a tray of instruments used for central venous cannulation. A manikin simulates a patient in traumatic shock.

(5 minute station)

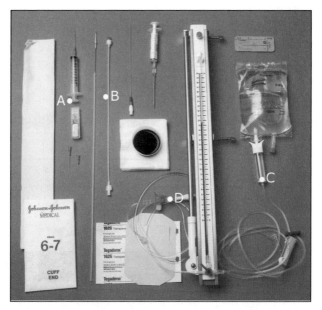

fig 4.20

1 Name the items labelled A, B, C and D.

2 Demonstrate the siting, introduction and confirming of the position of a central venous catheter on the manikin.

Answers

(A)   (C)

(B)   (D)

STATION 4.21

Treatment

Please tick the appropriate column in the following questions.

(5 minute station)

	True	False
1 The indications for diagnostic peritoneal lavage in blunt abdominal trauma are:		
(a) Unexplained hypotension	☐	☐
(b) Abdominal distension	☐	☐
(c) A 'silent' abdomen	☐	☐
(d) Abdominal skin bruising	☐	☐

2 The instruments in fig 4.21a are set out for diagnostic peritoneal lavage.

Name those labelled A, B, C, D and E.

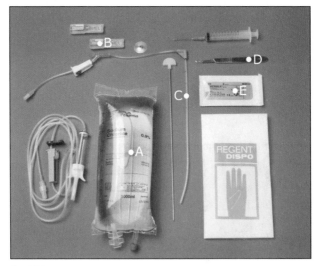

fig 4.21a

Answers

(A)   (D)

(B)   (E)

(C)

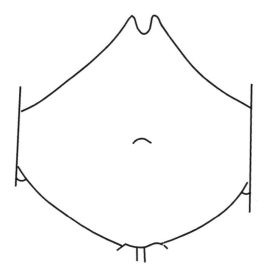

fig 4.21b

3 In the diagram of the abdomen above, choose the site most commonly used for diagnostic peritoneal lavage.

Chapter 1:
Cardiovascular Diseases
and Haematology Answers

CHAPTER 1

Cardiovascular Diseases and Haematology Answers

STATION 1.1

Patient history

I am 43 years old and have had Type 2 dependent diabetes for the past four years. I have had raised blood pressure for the last three years. About six months ago I began to experience a dull aching in the front of my chest, particularly when running or 'overstraining'. The pains last from 3 to 5 minutes but then settle down. In the last month the pain has been coming on more regularly and I have had two episodes of pain while at rest.

This episode of pain began 6 – 8 hours ago while I was watching television. It is the worst pain I've ever had, like someone sitting on my chest. The pain is across the front of my chest and radiates to my jaw and left arm. The pain is not related to position or breathing. It was eased with oxygen in the ambulance and with some spray under my tongue in the Emergency Department.

My father died aged 62 of heart problems. My older brother also has heart disease (angina). I am really worried that this is heart pain but surely I am far too young.

I have smoked about 10–20 cigarettes a day since I was 17 and drink 2–3 whiskies at night. I do not know my cholesterol level, but am otherwise well.

Assessment	Good	Adequate	Poor/not done
1 Appropriate introduction (full name and role)	☐	☐	☐
2 Explains purpose of interview	☐	☐	☐
3 Establishes previous history of similar chest pain	☐	☐	☐
4 Establishes onset of current chest pain		☐	☐
5 Establishes character of pain		☐	☐
6 Establishes site of the pain		☐	☐

7 Establishes sites of radiation of the pain ☐ ☐

8 Establishes relieving factors ☐ ☐ ☐

9 Establishes exacerbating factors ☐ ☐ ☐

10 Establishes associated factors
(eg palpitations, sweating, nausea,
dyspnoea) ☐ ☐ ☐

11 Establishes associated risk
factors of ischaemic disease:

Smoking ☐ ☐

Hypertension ☐ ☐

Diabetes ☐ ☐

History of IHD, PVD, Stroke ☐ ☐

Family history of IHD, Stroke ☐ ☐

Alcohol excess ☐ ☐

Hyperlipidaemia ☐ ☐

12 Elicits patient's concerns and responds
sensitively ☐ ☐ ☐

13 Appropriate questioning technique ☐ ☐ ☐

14 Summarises history back to patient ☐ ☐ ☐

15 Systematic, organised approach ☐ ☐ ☐

16 Makes the correct diagnosis ☐ ☐ ☐

SP to Mark

17 This doctor was empathic ☐ ☐ ☐

Diagnosis
Ischaemic cardiac chest pain – unstable angina/myocardial infarction

STATION 1.2

Patient history

I am 29 years old and a policeman. I am normally fit and well and have no significant illnesses of note. I do not smoke or drink alcohol. Over the last week I thought I had flu, with worsening lethargy, muscle pain and a sore throat. In the last two days I have also had a fever and chest pain.

The pain is sharp, in the middle of my chest and it radiates to my shoulders and the left side of my chest. The pain seems to be worse when I am lying down but seems better when I lean forward. It is also eased with paracetamol or aspirin. I've never had anything like this. It feels like a heart attack but I'm far too young for something like that.

Assessment	Good	Adequate	Poor/not done
1 Appropriate introduction (full name and role)	☐	☐	☐
2 Explains purpose of interview	☐	☐	☐
3 Establishes any previous similar episodes of pain	☐	☐	☐
4 Establishes onset of the chest pain		☐	☐
5 Establishes character of the chest pain		☐	☐
6 Establishes site of the pain		☐	☐
7 Establishes radiation of the pain		☐	☐
8 Establishes exacerbating factors (eg position)		☐	☐
9 Establishes relieving factors		☐	☐
10 Establishes associated symptoms (eg fever, pharyngitis, myalgia)	☐	☐	☐
11 Excludes risk factors of ischaemic heart disease	☐	☐	☐
12 Elicits patient's concerns and responds sensitively	☐	☐	☐
13 Appropriate questioning technique	☐	☐	☐
14 Avoids or explains jargon	☐	☐	☐

15 Summarises history back to patient,
    including concerns ☐ ☐ ☐

16 Systematic, organised approach ☐ ☐ ☐

17 Makes a reasonable attempt
    at the diagnosis ☐ ☐ ☐

Diagnosis
Acute viral pericarditis

Comment
Acute pericarditis is inflammation of the pericardium. It is characterised clinically by a sharp anterior chest pain, eased with leaning forward and NSAIDs, and exacerbated by lying down, movement and inspiration. The pain may radiate to the shoulders, neck and back.

Principal causes:

- **bacterial**: *Streptococcus*, *Staphylococcus*, *Haemophilus*, tuberculosis
- **viral**: this is a common cause; Coxsackie may occur in epidemics
- **metabolic**: uraemia
- **malignancy**: bronchial, breast, leukaemia, myeloma, Hodgkin's disease
- **post-myocardial infarction**: common after anterior MIs
- **Dressler's syndrome**: occurs one month to one year after an acute MI. It is an autoimmune disorder characterised by fever, pericarditis and pericardial effusion.

STATION 1.3a

Counselling

I am 33 years old and have previously been fit and well. My father died unexpectedly six weeks ago of a heart attack. In the last 3 – 4 weeks I have been experiencing left sided chest pains and I am worried that these might be angina.

The pain is just below my nipple and is sharp in nature. It seems to go through to my back and is made worse when I press on the area where the pain is. The pain lasts a few seconds at a time and then stops. There is no association with exertion and I have no other symptoms with it. I have never suffered similar pains in the past.

I have smoked 15 – 20 cigarettes a day for 10 years and drink 20 – 30 units of alcohol per week, mainly in the form of beer. I am not diabetic and I have not had any heart problems, a stroke or blood vessel disease. There is no other family history of heart disease, diabetes or stroke. At school I was a keen sportsman but have let myself go recently. I now do little exercise; I know I am overweight. I am not taking any medications.

I am very concerned about the pains and think I may be in danger of having a heart attack, like my father. I think perhaps I should consider changing my lifestyle.

Assessment	Good	Adequate	Poor/not done
1 Appropriate introduction (full name and role)	☐	☐	☐
2 Explains purpose of interview	☐	☐	☐
3 Establishes chest pains only started after father's death	☐	☐	☐
4 Establishes characteristics of the pain:			
Site		☐	☐
Character		☐	☐
Duration		☐	☐
Radiation		☐	☐
Relieving factors		☐	☐
Exacerbating factors		☐	☐
Associated symptoms	☐	☐	☐

5 Establishes patient's risk factors for
ischaemic heart disease:

Smoking □ □

Alcohol intake □ □

Lipids □ □

Family history of IHD, Stroke, PVD □ □

Previous medical history, eg diabetes,
PVD, IHD, Stroke □ □

6 Elicits patient's concerns and
responds sensitively □ □ □

7 Reassures patient of benign
nature of chest pain □ □ □

8 Appropriate questioning technique □ □ □

9 Avoids or explains jargon □ □ □

10 Summarises history back to patient,
including concerns □ □ □

11 Signals change in focus of interview,
towards discussion of risk factors/lifestyle
changes □ □ □

12 Clearly addresses main areas where change
is possible (smoking, exercise, diet) □ □ □

13 Works collaboratively with patient to set
goals (encourages a dialogue) □ □ □

14 Offers appropriate support
(smoking counsellor, dietician) □ □ □

15 Checks whether patient has any questions □ □ □

16 Systematic, organised approach □ □ □

SP to Mark

17 This doctor was non-judgemental □ □ □

18 I found it easy to talk to the doctor □ □ □

Diagnosis
Non-ischaemic chest pain probably of musculoskeletal origin

STATION 1.4

Patient history

I am 67 years old and I have had angina for eight years. I have not had a heart attack. In the last 2 – 3 months I have been getting fast, irregular palpitations. I am not aware of anything that specifically brings them on. When I get them, I also feel a tightness across my chest, not unlike my normal angina, with dizziness, sweating, nausea and a feeling that I am going to pass out. I have never lost consciousness. The palpitations last between 30 seconds and 5 minutes and have, on occasion, woken me up.

I am known to have heart problems but have no diabetes, blood vessel disease in my legs or feet and have not had a stroke. I gave up smoking six years ago and drink 5 – 6 gin and tonics per week. I am on aspirin and GTN spray. I am frightened about what might be going on and whether this means my heart problem is getting worse.

Assessment	Good	Adequate	Poor/not done
1 Appropriate introduction (full name and role)	☐	☐	☐
2 Establishes duration of the symptoms	☐	☐	☐
3 Establishes character of the palpitations (ie rate and rhythm)	☐	☐	☐
4 Establishes onset and duration of the palpitations	☐	☐	☐
5 Establishes/excludes associated symptoms:			
Sweating		☐	☐
Fainting		☐	☐
Dizziness		☐	☐
Loss of consciousness		☐	☐
Chest pain		☐	☐
Nausea		☐	☐

6 Establishes risk factors for cardiac disease and palpitations:

Smoking ☐ ☐

Alcohol excess ☐ ☐

IHD, Stroke, PVD ☐ ☐

Diabetes ☐ ☐

Hypertension ☐ ☐

7 Establishes present medications:

Aspirin and GTN spray ☐ ☐ ☐

8 Elicits patient's concerns and responds
   sensitively ☐ ☐ ☐

9 Appropriate questioning technique ☐ ☐ ☐

10 Avoids or explains jargon ☐ ☐ ☐

11 Summarises history back to patient,
   including concerns ☐ ☐ ☐

12 Systematic, organised approach ☐ ☐ ☐

Diagnosis

Paroxysmal fast irregular palpitations – differential includes paroxysmal atrial fibrillation or ventricular tachyarrhythmia

STATION 1.5

Patient history

I am a retired chartered surveyor, aged 63. I was well until eight months ago, when I started to experience shortness of breath when walking. Initially it didn't worry me too much, and I could still walk 3 – 4 miles on the flat. However, in the last few months this has progressively worsened and now I can only manage 400 – 500 metres, and less on hills. I am forced to stop because of the breathlessness. In the last 3 – 4 weeks my ankles have been swelling to the point where I can no longer put on my shoes. During this time I have had to sleep with three pillows. In the last few weeks I have woken several times with breathlessness, which has resolved about 10 minutes after I have got out of bed.

I have not had any palpitations, chest pain, cough, sputum, coughing up of blood or wheeziness.

I have never previously been ill, in particular I have never had any form of heart disease, a stroke, diabetes or blood vessel disease in my legs or feet. I gave up smoking 15 years ago, and drink only 1 – 2 pints of beer per week. I am not on any medications at present. I am feeling quite distressed about what is happening. I only retired recently and my wife and I had lots of travel plans, but I can't imagine doing much at all, feeling like this.

Assessment	Good	Adequate	Poor/not done
1 Appropriate introduction (full name and role)	☐	☐	☐
2 Establishes the duration of symptoms	☐	☐	☐
3 Establishes previous and present exercise tolerance	☐	☐	☐
4 Establishes presence of peripheral oedema	☐	☐	☐
5 Establishes three pillow orthopnoea and episodes of paroxysmal nocturnal dyspnoea	☐	☐	☐
6 Excludes other cardiac symptoms (eg palpitations, angina)	☐	☐	☐
7 Excludes respiratory symptoms (eg cough, sputum, wheeze, haemoptysis)	☐	☐	☐

8 Excludes common precipitating causes
and risk factors for heart failure:

Ischaemic heart disease ☐ ☐

Hypertension ☐ ☐

Alcohol excess ☐ ☐

Smoking ☐ ☐

Valvular heart disease ☐ ☐

Current medications ☐ ☐

Known diabetes, stroke or
peripheral vascular disease ☐ ☐

9 Elicits patient's concerns and responds
sensitively ☐ ☐ ☐

10 Appropriate questioning technique ☐ ☐ ☐

11 Avoids or explains jargon ☐ ☐ ☐

12 Summarises history back to patient,
including concerns ☐ ☐ ☐

13 Systematic, organised approach ☐ ☐ ☐

SP to Mark

14 The doctor was empathic ☐ ☐ ☐

Diagnosis
Idiopathic cardiac failure

STATION 1.6

Assessment	Good	Adequate	Poor/not done
1 Appropriate introduction (full name and role)	☐	☐	☐
2 Explains examination to patient and gains verbal consent	☐	☐	☐
3 Ensures patient is correctly positioned at 45°; chest is exposed	☐	☐	☐
4 Candidate washes their hands using the alcohol handwash provided (no marks if candidate only expresses the need to wash if handwash is provided)	☐	☐	☐
5 Observes patient from the end of the bed commenting on the wellbeing of the patient ie distressed/undistressed or well/unwell and then on the presence/absence of peripheral oedema, saphenous vein graft scars, signs of PVD; venous disease; ulceration; ascites; hepatomegaly; sternotomy/thoracotomy scar; mitral facies; anaemia	☐	☐	☐
6 Examines the hands – commenting on presence/absence of clubbing; stigmata of infective endocarditis; anaemia; tar staining; perfusion	☐	☐	☐
7 Examines the radial pulse – commenting on the rate; regularity; volume, symmetry and vessel wall	☐	☐	☐
8 Examines for collapsing pulse – **Examiner asks 'What are you doing?'** 'What does it represent?' (This is a sign of aortic regurgitation)	☐	☐	☐
9 Asks for, and comments on BP – absolute value and pulse pressure	☐	☐	☐

Answers

10 Examines the face commenting on presence/absence of anaemia; corneal arcus; xanthelasma; mitral facies; central cyanosis ☐   ☐   ☐

11 Examines the carotid pulses – commenting on symmetry and character ☐   ☐   ☐

12 Assesses the JVP – commenting on the height above angle of Louis and waveform; attempts to augment ☐   ☐   ☐

13 Re-examines and comments on presence/absence of sternotomy scar/lateral thoracotomy scar ☐   ☐   ☐

14 Palpates for apex beat defining position and character ☐   ☐   ☐

15 Palpates correctly and comments on the presence/absence of a left parasternal heave and thrills ☐   ☐   ☐

16 Auscultates for murmurs with appropriate use of bell and diaphragm in all four cardiac areas ☐   ☐   ☐

17 Correctly auscultates for mitral murmurs with patient turned on their left ☐   ☐   ☐

18 Correctly auscultates for aortic stenosis with radiation to carotid pulses ☐   ☐   ☐

19 Correctly auscultates for aortic regurgitation with patient leaning forward/in expiration ☐   ☐   ☐

20 Auscultates the lung bases and comments on presence/absence of signs of heart failure ☐   ☐   ☐

21 Palpates and comments on presence/absence of sacral oedema ☐   ☐   ☐

22 Repositions patient to ensure dignity and comfort; thanks patient ☐   ☐   ☐

23 Completes examination by asking
    for dipstix urine (urinalysis); palpation
    of peripheral pulses; auscultation for aortic,
    renal and femoral bruits ☐ ☐ ☐

24 Presents findings in a logical and
    appropriate manner ☐ ☐ ☐

25 Is able to present an appropriate
    differential diagnosis; causes and
    complications ☐ ☐ ☐

Answers

STATION 1.7

Assessment	Good	Adequate	Poor/not done
1 Appropriate introduction (full name and role)	☐	☐	☐
2 Explains examination to patient; gains verbal consent	☐	☐	☐
3 Ensures patient is comfortable; correctly positioned at 45°; chest exposed	☐	☐	☐
4 Candidate washes their hands using the alcohol handwash provided (no marks if candidate only expresses the need to wash if handwash is provided)	☐	☐	☐
5 Stands at the end of the bed – observes and comments on the wellbeing of the patient and then on the presence/absence of peripheral oedema; saphenous vein graft scar; signs of PVD; venous disease; ulceration; ascites; hepatomegaly; sternotomy; mitral facies; anaemia	☐	☐	☐
6 Examines the carotid pulses – commenting on symmetry and character			
7 Assesses the JVP – commenting on height above manubriosternal angle and wave form; attempts to augment	☐	☐	☐
8 Examines and comments on the apex beat defining position and character	☐	☐	☐
9 Examines and comments on the presence/ absence of heaves and thrills	☐	☐	☐
10 Auscultates in all four cardiac areas with appropriate use of bell and diaphragm	☐	☐	☐
11 With patient lying on their left side – specifically examines for mitral stenosis with bell	☐	☐	☐

12 Specifically examines for mitral
    regurgitation, listening at the axilla   ☐   ☐   ☐

13 Specifically examines for aortic stenosis
    listening for radiation into the carotids   ☐   ☐   ☐

14 Specifically examines for aortic
    regurgitation at lower left sternal edge
    with patient leaning forward in expiration   ☐   ☐   ☐

15 Listens at the lung bases commenting
    on presence/absence of signs of heart
    failure   ☐   ☐   ☐

16 Feels for sacral oedema   ☐   ☐   ☐

17 Repositions patient to ensure dignity and
    comfort; thanks patient   ☐   ☐   ☐

18 Finishes examination by requesting
    urinalysis, examination of peripheral
    pulses; blood pressure; bruits – aortic;
    renal and femoral   ☐   ☐   ☐

19 Presents findings in a fluent, logical
    manner   ☐   ☐   ☐

20 Presents an appropriate differential
    diagnosis; causes and complications   ☐   ☐   ☐

Answers

STATION 1.8

Assessment	Good	Adequate	Poor/not done
1 Appropriate introduction (full name and role)	☐	☐	☐
2 Explains procedure to patient; gains verbal consent	☐	☐	☐
3 Correctly places sphygmomanometer cuff around patient's arm using correct sized cuff for patient	☐	☐	☐
4 Candidate washes their hands using the alcohol handwash provided (no marks if candidate only expresses the need to wash if handwash is provided)	☐	☐	☐
5 Examiner asks, 'What would happen to the BP results if the cuff is too small?' (Answer – the reading is **falsely** elevated and vice versa for too large a cuff)	☐	☐	☐
6 Palpates and locates radial pulse	☐	☐	☐
7 Inflates then deflates cuff to estimate systolic pressure	☐	☐	☐
8 Palpates and locates brachial pulse and places stethoscope diaphragm over pulse	☐	☐	☐
9 Reinflates cuff (whilst listening to pulse) to just above systolic pressure	☐	☐	☐
10 Deflates cuff at an appropriate rate	☐	☐	☐
11 Correctly gives systolic and diastolic values to within 5 mmHg	☐	☐	☐
12 Examiner asks:			
(a) What is the pulse pressure in this case? Is this normal? (normal 120–80 = 40 mmHg)	☐	☐	☐
(b) How else may you take the BP and why?	☐	☐	☐

Correct answers:

	Good	adequate	Poor/not done
(i) Lying/ standing for postural drop	☐	☐	☐
(ii) In both arms – for symmetry	☐	☐	☐
13 Examiner invites student to explain results to patient. Candidate explains results correctly in an appropriate manner	☐	☐	☐
14 Thanks patient and ensures they are comfortable.	☐	☐	☐

STATION 1.9

Assessment	Good	adequate	Poor/not done
1 Appropriate introduction (full name and role)	☐	☐	☐
2 Explains examination to patient; gains verbal consent	☐	☐	☐
3 Ensures patient is correctly positioned at 45°; chest exposed	☐	☐	☐
4 Candidate washes their hands using the alcohol handwash provided (no marks if candidate only expresses the need to wash if handwash is provided)	☐	☐	☐
5 Correctly lifts patient's chin and asks them to look across to their left	☐	☐	☐
6 Examiner asks, 'Show me where you are looking for the JVP' (Correct – between the two heads of sternomastoid on a line running up to the angle of the jaw to the ear lobe)	☐	☐	☐
7 Examiner asks, 'Show me how you would estimate the height' (Correct – vertical height above manubriosternal angle)	☐	☐	☐
8 Examiner asks, 'How can you augment the JVP?' (Correct – push on abdomen/ liver to demonstrate abdominojugular/ hepatojugular reflex)	☐	☐	☐

9 **Examiner asks, 'How can you differentiate the JVP from the carotid pulse?'** ☐ ☐ ☐

(Correct –

(a) JVP – double wave form; carotid – single pulsation ☐ ☐

(b) JVP – Obstructed – augmented at base of neck ☐ ☐

(c) JVP – augmented with abdominojugular reflex ☐ ☐

(d) Carotid pulse is palpable single pulsation ☐ ☐

10 **Examiner asks, 'Show me what you would do if you thought the JVP was 'very high', (Correct – student sits patient upright at 90 degrees; likewise if JVP very low – lie patient down)'** ☐ ☐ ☐

11 Covers patient ensuring comfort and dignity; thanks patient ☐ ☐ ☐

STATION 1.10

Assessment	Good	Adequate	Poor/not done
1 Appropriate introduction (full name and role)	☐	☐	☐
Colour, skin nutrition and warmth. Muscle bulk. Technique of palpation and description of peripheral pulses (ie femoral, popliteal, posterior tibial, dorsalis pedis, peroneal)	☐	☐	☐
2 Measurement of brachial systolic pressure		☐	☐
Measurement of ankle systolic pressure		☐	☐
Calculation of the pressure index	☐	☐	☐
3 Does all in a fluent, professional manner	☐	☐	☐

Comment

Chronic lower limb ischaemia clinically manifests as trophic skin change and reduction in muscle bulk. Reduced or abnormal femoral pulses suggest aorto-iliac disease; the abdomen should be palpated to exclude an aneurysm.

Ankle: brachial pressure index is a sensitive measure of foot perfusion. The post-exercise index is measured after 1 – 5 minutes exercising on a treadmill. It indicates the extent of collateral circulation and the degree of occlusive disease. In significant disease the index falls following exercise.

STATION 1.11

Assessment	Good	Adequate	Poor/not done
1 Ulcer: establishes:			
Site, size	☐	☐	☐
Flat/sloping edge	☐	☐	☐
Slough-covered base with no granulation	☐	☐	☐
No deep penetration	☐	☐	☐
Surrounding induration and pigmentation	☐	☐	☐
2 Additional history:			
Pain and disability	☐	☐	☐
Varicose veins	☐	☐	☐
Previous DVT and trauma	☐	☐	☐
Peripheral vascular disease and diabetes	☐	☐	☐
3 Additional examination:			
Extent of induration		☐	☐
Fixation of ulcer		☐	☐
Ankle mobility		☐	☐
Inguinal lymphadenopathy		☐	☐
Venous incompetence		☐	☐
Pulses and sensation in the leg	☐	☐	☐
Abnormality of other leg	☐	☐	☐
4 Carries out all in a fluent, professional manner	☐	☐	☐

Comment

Venous ulceration is a late sequela of the post-phlebitic limb. The ulceration is sited just above the medial and, to a lesser extent, the lateral malleolus. It can be large but rarely penetrates the deep tissues. Although it can be healed by elevation and reduction of swelling, it frequently persists, causing chronic discomfort and severe pain, particularly if accompanied by secondary infection. Recurrence frequently follows minor trauma. Venous bleeding can occasionally be quite severe, but is readily controlled by elevation and a firm dressing.

Other common causes of leg ulceration include trauma and chronic ischaemia. In the latter the ulceration occurs over and between the toes, and over pressure sites, particularly the heel and malleoli. The condition may co-exist with venous problems, and pulses must always be checked.

Diabetic ulcers may be ischaemic but an associated peripheral neuropathy places the foot at risk of ulceration, particularly over weight-bearing areas, such as the heads of the metatarsals. The problem is accentuated by the predisposition to infection. With all lower limb ulcers, carefully examine and monitor progress of the skin edge for evidence of malignancy. Malignant change in a pre-existing ulcer, or primary malignancy can be easily missed when sited over classical sites for other pathology.

STATION 1.12

Assessment	Good	Adequate	Poor/not done
1 Appropriate introduction (full name and role)	☐	☐	☐
2 Explains procedure and gains verbal consent	☐	☐	☐
3 Ensure the patient is lying comfortably on a bed sitting at 45°. Expose the full length of both legs, the patient being in underwear	☐	☐	☐
4 Candidate washes their hands using the alcohol handwash provided (no marks if candidate only expresses the need to wash if handwash is provided)	☐	☐	☐
5 Briefly comment on the normal nutrition of the feet, ie no peripheral oedema, normal colour, nails, skin – no skin changes	☐	☐	☐
6 **Examiner asks – 'Show me how and where you are going to feel for the femoral pulses'**			
Answer – Site just below the inguinal ligament at the mid-inguinal point (midway between the anterior, superior, iliac spine and the symphysis pubis – midline) compressing the artery onto the head of the femur with three longitudinal placed fingers			
7 Examines and comments on femoral pulses one at a time then compares the two sides. Comments on the presence, the rate, the regularity, volume and symmetry of the two sides	☐	☐	☐

8 Examine popliteal pulses individually
   and compares – compresses the distal
   popliteal onto the back of the upper end
   of the tibia with the tips of the fingers
   from both ends wrapped around the
   upper leg compressing between the heads
   of the gastrocnemis, subject's leg being
   slightly flexed. It is easier to do this sitting
   on the bed (a Sister not usually being
   present to condemn this habit!). Comments
   on the presence of symmetry   ☐   ☐   ☐

9 Examines for dorsalis pedis arteries – along
   a line from the mid-anterior point between
   the malleoli and the first digital web
   compressing on the bones of the tarsus.   ☐   ☐   ☐

10 Examines for posterior tibial arteries.
   Compresses the artery onto the medial
   talus behind and just below the medial
   malleolus. Comments on presence and
   symmetry   ☐   ☐   ☐

11 A perforating peroneal artery maybe
   palpated anterior to the lateral malleolus.
   Looked for the end of previous examination
   if one of the foot pulses is weak or absent
   (congenitally or from disease)   ☐   ☐   ☐

12 Listens with stethoscope over both femoral
   arteries and adductor hiatus medial
   aspect both thighs a hands- breadth
   above the knee   ☐   ☐   ☐

13 Ensures dignity, covers and comfort and
   thanks them   ☐   ☐   ☐

14 Presents a summary of the findings in a
   fluent and logical manner   ☐   ☐   ☐

15 Correctly identifies any pathology present.   ☐   ☐   ☐

STATION 1.13

Assessment	Good	Adequate	Poor/not done
1 Appropriate introduction (full name and role)	☐	☐	☐
2 Explains examination of his foot, leg and pulses and gains verbal consent	☐	☐	☐
3 Ensures patient is lying comfortably. Removes sheets and bed cradle and knee overlying paper towel	☐	☐	☐
4 Candidate washes their hands using the alcohol handwash provided (no marks if candidate only expresses the need to wash if handwash is provided)	☐	☐	☐
5 Asks the patient how long the lesion has been present, if it's getting bigger and is it painful and tender.	☐	☐	☐
6 Observes the ulcer from the side, if necessary the end and other side of the bed	☐	☐	☐
7 Comments on the site, the size, the shape, the edge, flat, punched out, undermined, raised, everted or list; the floor – depth, covering, discharge, penetration, fistulation, surrounding induration, swelling, colour	☐	☐	☐
8 Gently examines between all toes over both malleoli of both legs then carefully raises both legs to examine heels and foot colour changes on elevation	☐	☐	☐
9 With help turns the patient so he is sitting on the side of the bed, thus allowing the legs to become dependent. Observes and comments on the number of seconds taken for return of normal colour and any reactive hyperaemia	☐	☐	☐

10 Repositions patient in bed and examines
all pulses (as in previous station).
Comments on the presence/ absence
of both sets of femoral, popliteal,
dorsalis pedis and posterior tibial pulses ☐ ☐ ☐

11 Looks for scars, nail changes and
amputations. Moves to observe from
end of the bed ☐ ☐ ☐

12 Examines along the midline above the
umbilicus for presence of abdominal
aortic aneurysm ☐ ☐ ☐

13 Attempts to auscultate for aortic,
femoral and renal bruits. Examiner to stop
candidate. 'Please continue' ☐ ☐ ☐

14 Ensures towel is placed over ulcer and
replacement of cradle and bed clothes
ensuring dignity and comfort.
Thanks patient ☐ ☐ ☐

15 Presents findings in a fluent, logical
manner ☐ ☐ ☐

STATION 1.14

1 I normal	II normal	III normal	IV C
2 I normal	II normal	III raised	IV A
3 I raised	II raised	III raised	IV F
4 I raised	II raised	III raised	IV B
5 I normal	II raised	III raised	IV E
6 I normal	II raised	III raised	IV D

Comment

Acute bleeding disorders encountered during surgery or in its immediate aftermath are due to haemodilution from IV fluids or large volume banked blood transfusions. Other causes are hypoxia, intravascular haemolysis, infection and thrombosis. Abruptio placentae, amniotic fluid embolus and retained products of conception produce bleeding disorders in obstetric practice.

The investigation of a suspected bleeding tendency begins with the bleeding history, this may suggest an acquired or congenital disorder of primary or secondary haemostasis. Clinical evaluation of the patient's history, family history, details of site, frequency and character of haemorrhagic manifestations (eg purpura, bruising, haematoma, haemarthrosis) may suggest the diagnosis, this is confirmed by screening tests and, if necessary, by specific investigations.

STATION 1.15

1 (C) (d)

G6PD deficiency is an X-linked disorder which has several recognised variants. The variant suffered by black Africans and black African Americans (G6PD GdA-) has a self-limiting haemolytic anaemia as the bone marrow is able to compensate by increasing red cell production.

However, in the Mediterranean variant (G6PD Gd Med) following an oxidant insult (eg sepsis, myocardial infarction or diabetic coma) gross haemolysis occurs and will be fatal unless the cause is treated and the patient is transfused. Classically this reaction may be seen after the ingestion of fava beans. Heinz bodies are seen in the blood film (hence the expression, 'Beans means Heinz'!).

2 (D) (e)

This patient presents with the classical symptoms of a mycoplasma pneumonia. This is associated with a cold antibody (IgM) Coombs' positive autoimmune haemolytic anaemia. A Coombs' test is performed using a combination of the patient's serum and Coomb's serum.

Coombs' serum is an antihuman serum and causes agglutination of the patient's red cells if certain antibodies are present on their surface. The temperature at which these antibodies attach themselves to the red cells characterise the haemolysis into cold (37 °C) and warm (40 °C) types.

3 (B) (c)

This patient has β-thalassaemia which is a common haemolytic disorder especially found around the Mediterranean, the Middle East and the Indian sub-continent. The patients with severe disease, thalassaemia major, present in the first few years of life with recurrent infections, severe anaemia and extramedullary haemopoiesis. These patients require regular transfusion and often develop transfusion siderosis. This is countered by using the chelating agent desferrioxamine.

4 (E) (a)

SLE is associated with a warm (IgG) Coombs' positive autoimmune haemolytic anaemia. Other causes include carcinoma, haematological malignancy (eg CLL and lymphoma) and drugs, the most common being methyl dopa.

5 (A) (b)

Sickle cell disease is a common haemolytic disorder in black races particularly those from Africa, the Caribbean and in African Americans. It also occurs in the Indian sub-continent and the Middle East. The haemolysis is often mild in heterozygotes and may remain undiscovered until a severe insult, such as sepsis or general anaesthesia. Homozygotes present in childhood and suffer a debilitating multisystem disorder. Complications include bone pain, bone necrosis, including avascular necrosis of the femoral head, and rarely *Salmonella* osteomyelitis; cerebral infarcts and epilepsy, acute papillary necrosis and tubulointerstitial nephritis causing renal failure and pneumonitis leading to respiratory failure.

Treatment of an acute sickle cell crisis should include treatment of the precipitating cause, maintenance of hydration with intravenous fluids, oxygen via face mask and analgesia, usually with opiates.

STATION 1.16

(1) E   (4) F

(2) C   (5) B

(3) A   (6) D

Comment

Warfarin is a coumarin anticoagulant which exerts its effects by acting as a vitamin K antagonist, inhibiting factors II, VII, IX and X of the clotting cascade. Warfarin therapy should aim to maintain the INR between 2 – 3 for thromboembolic disease and between 3 – 4 for prosthetic heart valves. One should never reverse the effects of warfarin with a full dose of vitamin K (10 mg) unless instructed to do so by a haematologist or senior medical opinion. If a full dose is given the patient cannot be anticoagulated with warfarin for three months and therefore requires subcutaneous heparin. If the patient is actively bleeding the anticoagulant effect can be reversed using FFP and small doses of vitamin K, 1 – 4 mg.

When faced with a patient with liver disease who has a raised INR, vitamin K should be administered carefully by intravenous injection. These patients should not receive intramuscular injections as this causes severe intramuscular haematomas and necrosis.

STATION 1.17

Blood test	Blood bottle
(1) Check Hb post transfusion	A
(2) Blood glucose	B or F
(3) Serum lipids	B
(4) Cross match	D
(5) Serum potassium	B
(6) Autoantibody screen	B
(7) Malaria screen	A
(8) Atypical pneumonia screen	B
(9) Thyroid function tests	B
(10) Platelet count – thrombocytopenia	A

(11) INR	C
(12) Amylase	B
(13) FDPs (fibrinogen degradation products)	C
(14) Serum osmolality	B
(15) ESR	A or E

Bottle

A – 4.5 ml bottle containing EDTA. Traditionally has purple top. Principally used for FBC; glycosylated Hb (HbAlc), blood film and T-cell and B-cell markers. It is now used for ESR.

B – This is a 7 ml bottle containing a clot activating agent (gel) in its base. It is used for U+Es, serum glucose, amylase, LFTs, TFTs, lipids, cardiac enzymes, autoantibodies and osmolality. It may have an orange or an orange and black speckled top.

C – This is a 4.5 ml bottle containing sodium citrate. It is used for coagulation tests including INR, APTT, TT, FDPs and D-Dimer. It has a light blue top.

D – This is a 7.0 ml bottle with a pink top which is solely used for cross match samples. It has to be completed including a signature.

E – This black topped bottle is used for an ESR but has been largely replaced by the FBC bottle.

F – This grey topped bottle is used solely for measurement of serum glucose. Its use has been made redundant in most hospitals due to the ability of the new machines to analyse glucose from bottle B.

STATION 1.18

1 (D) 5 (A)

2 (G) 6 (C)

3 (F) 7 (E)

4 (B)

Comment

Creatine phosphokinase (CPK) or creatine kinase has several isoenzymes and is found primarily in voluntary muscle, myocardium and brain tissue. Medical students are often only aware that a raised CPK or CK is caused by an acute myocardial infarction. However, strokes, recurrent falls, non-accidental injury and myositis are all common causes and need to be taken into consideration in a differential diagnosis. Patients should not be given thrombolytic therapy solely on the basis of a raised CPK.

STATION 1.19

1 For limb leads see fig 1A, page XX; for chest leads V1–V6 see fig 1.19

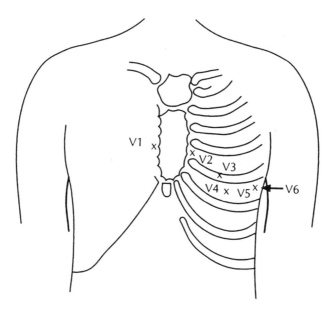

2   (a) Sinus bradycardia, 56 bpm

    (b) Sinus rhythm

    (c) Normal axis

    (d) No the P wave is broadened and notched suggesting P mitrale

    (e) Yes

    (f) Yes

    (g) ST elevation: leads II, III and aVF

       ST depression: leads V3–6, I and aVL

       This is consistent with an acute inferior MI with widespread septolateral ischaemia.

STATION 1.20

1 (a) True (b) True (c) False (d) False (e) False

This ECG shows a right bundle branch block pattern with first degree heart block and left axis deviation. This combination is termed trifascicular block. The rate is approximately 100 bpm. This pattern may lead to complete heart block and the patient should have a 24-hour tape to exclude prolonged episodes of heart block. Such patients need a permanent pacemaker.

2 (a) True (b) True (c) False (d) True (e) False

This is a left bundle branch block pattern. There is a sinus tachycardia with P pulmonale. The axis is normal. Left bundle branch block is a pathological pattern whereas right bundle branch block occurs in approximately 3% of the healthy population.

3 (a) True (b) False (c) False (d) True (e) True

This patient is in atrial fibrillation. Rate:100–150; axis normal; voltage criteria of left ventricular hypertrophy – the S wave in V2 + the R wave in V5 > 40 mm. (In this case the SV1 + RV5 = 25 + 27 = 52 mm)

4 (a) True (b) True (c) False (d) True (e) True

The ECG shows an acute inferoposterior MI with lateral ischaemia. There is evidence of first degree heart block and such ischaemia predisposes to various degrees of atrioventricular nodal block. The patient should be treated with aspirin and, if no contraindications, thrombolysis.

5 (a) True (b) False (c) False (d) False (e) True

This ECG was taken from a patient with a large pulmonary embolism. There is a sinus tachycardia with the axis deviating towards the right. There is a right bundle branch block pattern and the rarely seen S1,Q3,T3 pattern (ie a deep S wave in lead I, and a Q wave and inverted T wave in lead III).

STATION 1.21

1 (a) False (b) True (c) False (d) True (e) True
This well centred chest radiograph (as evidenced by the opposing clavicular heads) shows acute pulmonary oedema with blunting of the right costodiaphragmatic angle and fluid in the horizontal fissure. The cardiothoracic ration is normal and this suggests an acute cardiac cause such as a myocardial infarction or an arrhythmia. the underlying cause needs to be corrected and the patient should be given oxygen and IV diuretics.

2 (a) True (b) False (c) False (d) False (e) False
This chest radiograph shows evidence of chronic biventricular cardiac failure. The six signs of cardiac failure on a CXR are cardiomegaly, pleural effusions, fluid in the horizontal fissure, upper lobe blood diversion, Kerley B lines and interstitial oedema (classically giving the fluffy 'bat winging' appearance). Kerley B lines are small horizontal straight lines at the bases of lung fields and represent fluid between the interlobular septa and lymphatics (not present on this radiograph).

3 (a) False (b) False (c) True (d) True (e) True
This radiograph shows 'mitralisation' of the left heart border. There is cardiomegaly and loss of the left atrial appendage leading to a straight left heart border. Associated radiographic signs include enlarged pulmonary arteries and 'pruning' of the peripheral pulmonary markings, consistent with secondary pulmonary hypertension. The mitral valve may also be calcified.

4 (a) True (b) False (c) True (d) False (e) False
This radiograph shows a large globular heart consistent with a pericardial effusion. As an effusion enlarges it may constrict the heart to the point where it is unable to contract. This is termed cardiac tamponade. Clinical signs associated with tamponade, or a large effusion, include low volume pulse, hypotension, pulsus paradoxus and Kussmaul's sign. The ECG shows small, low voltage complexes.

STATION 1.22

(A) Left main stem

(B) Right coronary artery

(C) Marginal branch of the right coronary artery

(D) Left anterior interventricular artery

(E) Apex of the left ventricle

(F) Stenosis in right coronary artery

1 Inferior leads II, III and aVF

2 Typically – sinus bradycardia and varying degrees of heart block including complete heart block. This may require insertion of a temporary pacemaker.

3 In symptomatic single vessel disease, balloon angioplasty is often recommended.

STATION 1.23

A 1 Carotid arteriogram/angiogram

    2 A – Common carotid artery
      B – Internal carotid artery
      C – External carotid artery

    3 Tight stenosis of the origin of the internal carotid artery

    4 Non-critical stenosis: aspirin or persantin therapy to reduce rouleaux formation and 3 to 6-monthly duplex scan surveillance

    Critical stenosis: balloon angioplasty or carotid endarterectomy

B				
1 (a) no	(b) no	(c) yes	(d) no
2 (a) yes	(b) no	(c) no	(d) yes
3 (a) no	(b) yes	(c) yes	(d) yes
4 (a) yes	(b) yes	(c) yes	(d) no

Comment
Atheromatous plaques in the intima may produce luminal narrowing or may ulcerate, producing atheromatous emboli, leading to a stroke. Critical stenosis (narrowing > 70%) or ulceration on angiography with TIAs requires revascularisation to restore normal blood flow to the cerebral hemisphere.

Answers

STATION 1.24

1   (a) Femoral angiogram (arteriogram)

    (b) Stenosis of the iliac arteries

    (c) Smoking, hypercholesterolaemia, diabetes mellitus, hypertension, family history of arterial disease

    (d) Claudication, rest pain, peripheral gangrene

2   (a) False   (b) True   (c) False   (d) False

Comment
Claudication is the main symptom of PVD, with rest pain and gangrene being the end result of disease progression. Angiography is indicated for progressive disease to ascertain suitability for vascular reconstruction. Long-term graft patency is also dependent on controlling or eliminating predisposing factors, such as diabetes, hypercholesterolaemia and smoking.

STATION 1.25

I am 47 years old and unemployed. I was admitted five days ago with newly diagnosed unstable angina and diabetes. I don't really understand what is going on despite the educational sessions from the specialist cardiac and diabetes nurses. I am particularly concerned about:

(1) When to take the spray?

(2) Will the spray fit in my hand bag?

(3) Will my angina stop me going to my keep fit classes?

Assessment	Good	Adequate	Poor/not done
1 Appropriate introduction (full name and role)	☐	☐	☐
2 Establishes patient understanding of GTN's use	☐	☐	☐
3 Explains situations in which to use the spray:			
Whenever angina pain comes on	☐	☐	☐
Prophylactically when you know pain may come on (eg before strenuous exertion)	☐	☐	☐
4 Explains in a clear, simple manner how to use the spray. Mentions the need to:	☐	☐	☐
Stop whatever you are doing and to sit down	☐	☐	☐
Shake the spray and then remove the top	☐	☐	☐
Give two sprays under the tongue	☐	☐	☐
If pain is unrelieved after 5 – 10 minutes, give two further sprays	☐	☐	☐
5 Warns that if pain is poorly relieved or unrelieved after 15 – 20 minutes take 300 mg of aspirin and call an ambulance	☐	☐	☐

6 Explains common side-effects
   (eg headache, dizziness and
   postural hypotension)   ☐   ☐   ☐

7 Invites questions and addresses
   patient's anxieties   ☐   ☐   ☐

8 Checks patient's understanding of
   information given to her   ☐   ☐   ☐

9 Systematic, organised approach   ☐   ☐   ☐

Answers

STATION 1.26

1 (A) Efferent arteriole   (H) Loop of Henlé

  (B) Afferent arteriole   (I) Ascending limb of the loop of Henlé

  (C) Bowman's capsule   (J) Distal convoluted tubule

  (D) Glomerulus   (K) Collecting duct

  (E) Cortex

  (F) Medulla

  (G) Descending limb of the loop of Henlé

2 (a) 4   (d) 3

  (b) 1   (e) 2

  (c) 2   (f) 1

Explanations

Site 1: ascending limb of the loop of Henlé. This is the site of action of loop diuretics, which inhibit resorption. They are extremely potent diuretics and cause hypokalaemia, hyponatraemia, hypomagnesaemia and postural hypotension.

Site 2: the proximal area of the distal convoluted tubule. This is the site of action of the thiazide diuretics bendrofluazide and metolazone. They inhibit sodium resorption and commonly cause hyponatraemia, hypokalaemia and hypomagnesaemia.

Site 3: the distal convoluted tubule. This is the site of action of potassium sparing diuretics such as amiloride and triamterene. These are weak diuretics but are used in combination with thiazides and loop diuretics.

Site 4: the collecting ducts. This is the site of action of the aldosterone antagonist spironolactone. This diuretic is principally used in the secondary hyperaldosteronism that occurs with cardiac, renal and hepatic failure.

STATION 1.27

1 (D) (e)
This patient describes two of the classical side-effects of amiodarone. This drug is useful in both supraventricular and ventricular arrhythmia but unfortunately has many side-effects. Patients should always be warned about the side-effects of the drug and this should be recorded in their notes. Common side-effects include: pulmonary fibrosis; photosensitive rash; slate grey pigmentation of the skin; derangement of the liver function tests; derangement of thyroid activity causing both hypo- and hyperthyroidism; microcorneal deposits.

2 (E) (a)
The patient describes a rare side-effect of digoxin; xanthopsia or the visual field turning yellow. Digoxin has a narrow therapeutic window and is a common cause of drug-induced side-effects, particularly in patients with impaired renal function. It commonly presents with bradycardia and nausea. It may cause both supraventricular and ventricular arrhythmias and, in high toxic levels, may require treatment with 'Digibind' which is a Fab fragment which binds to digoxin and makes it inert in the plasma.

3 (A) (f)
Shortness of breath post myocardial infarction may have many causes. Beta blockers have become established as one of the principal treatments during the initial 48 hours post-acute infarct but contraindications must be excluded viz asthma and moderate to severe heart failure.

4 (B) (c)
Calcium channel blockers are a common treatment for essential hypertension. The side-effects of flushing and headaches are due to vasodilatation. The other side-effect of fluid retention may cause worsening cardiac failure but may occur in isolation. Remember all ankle oedema is not due to cardiac failure!

5 (F) (b)
The medical treatment of Wolff–Parkinson–White includes flecainide and amiodarone which have a very similar side-effect profile. As when amiodarone is prescribed, the patient should be made aware of the common side-effects and this should be recorded in the notes.

6 (C) (d)
Sotalol is a class III anti-arrhythmic with partial beta blocker effect. It is a useful drug in the treatment of atrial fibrillation but cannot be used in patients with cardiac failure.

STATION 1.28

Patient history

I am 46 years old and work as a draftsman. I was taken to hospital after severe chest pain this morning and have been told that I've had a heart attack. I have been transferred from the Emergency Department for a 'clot busting' treatment. I have not been told anything more than this. I have been treated for high blood pressure and type 2 diabetes for the past seven years but have been otherwise well. I go to see the doctor in the diabetic clinic twice a year and have a few changes in the back of my eyes, which have remained unchanged in the past few years. I have never suffered with any bleeding problems or indigestion and have never been told that I have an ulcer. I have no other contraindications for thrombolysis treatment. I am a bit concerned when told about the risk of bleeding into the brain, but will have the treatment if you explain things carefully, but will not accept the therapy if I am not satisfied with your explanation.

Assessment	Good	Adequate	Poor/not done
1 Appropriate introduction (full name and role)	☐	☐	☐
2 Explains purpose of interview	☐	☐	☐
3 Establishes what patient has been told already about the treatement	☐	☐	☐
4 Clearly describes nature of treatment	☐	☐	☐
5 Mentions the common side-effects – flushing, warm feeling as the thrombolysis is given; dizziness; nausea and vomiting	☐	☐	☐
6 Mentions the uncommon side-effects:	☐	☐	☐
haemorrhagic stroke;	☐	☐	☐
gastrointestinal and general	☐	☐	☐
bleeding; severe allergic reaction:	☐	☐	☐
shortness of breath, wheeze and cardiovascular collapse	☐	☐	☐

7 Excludes absolute contraindications:

Active bleeding problems
(eg peptic ulceration) ☐ ☐

Streptokinase previously ☐ ☐

Major surgery within the last ten days ☐ ☐

Recent major trauma ☐ ☐

Any previous history of
intracranial haemorrhage ☐ ☐

Uncontrolled hypertension ☐ ☐

8 Discusses relative contraindications
(eg diabetic retinopathy) ☐ ☐ ☐

9 Invites questions and addresses
patient's concerns ☐ ☐ ☐

10 Checks patient's understanding
of information ☐ ☐ ☐

11 Systematic, organised approach ☐ ☐ ☐

SP to Mark

12 The doctor was empathic ☐ ☐ ☐

STATION 1.29

Comment

It is essential to make sure that when cross matching blood for a patient all the details are filled in correctly and as comprehensively as possible. Most mistakes related to blood transfusions are caused by bureaucratic error. The units of blood are collected from the blood bank with the lower part of the original request form, shown below. When putting up a new unit of blood, the unit details should be checked by two people, against the patient's details, and the details on the form below.

Answers

HEALTH AUTHORITY .... *ST. PETER'S* .... HOSPITAL

REQUEST FOR BLOOD FOR TRANSFUSION AND/OR GROUPING

Patient's surname	first name(s)	sex	date of birth	Ward/dept.	Hospital No.	Ethnic orig.
THOMAS	DEBRA	F	13/9/09	Flemming	123432	Caucasian

Consultant...... *DR LITTLE* .... Signature of doctor *Signature*
                                          making this request

Patient identified and blood taken by.. *CANDIDATE NAME* ...... at .*TIME*. hours on *(date)*.. *XX-MONTH-YEAR*

Clinical Diagnosis........ *MYELODYSPLASIA* .... Hb .*5.2*. g/dl.

Nature of operation or other reason for Transfusion ... *ANAEMIA* ....

Previous Transfusions?. *YES, MULTIPLE - last 2/52 ago* Group (if known) .*A Rh(+)*.

Reactions?...... *NIL* ....

Pregnancies?...... *NOT KNOWN* .... E.D.D. ....

Have Antibodies been reported?...... *NO* ....

REQUEST FOR:
Please tick or number box as appropriate

	Group Only *Serum will be kept for 7 days*
	packs immediately unchecked to save life ⎫
	packs urgent ⎬ *Telephone Hospital Blood Bank*
	packs whole for use at .... a.m./p.m. on................... ⎭
4 UNITS ✓	concentrated cells for use at .*A.S.A.P.*. a.m./*p.m* on.. *XX-MONTH-YEAR*

For other blood products telephone Hospital Blood Bank
Blood will be issued only if this form is properly completed and is accompanied by a correctly labelled specimen
of the patient's blood.

RECORD OF TRANSFUSION   Complete in ward. At end of transfusion affix to notes.

PATIENT'S BLOOD GROUP..... A ......   **RHESUS (D)**.. POSITIVE ......

The following packs are compatible with patient's serum **ANTIBODIES:**......................
                                          12 Noon
They will be returned to stock at........................ hours on (date) ..30.9.1998......

PACK NUMBER	GROUP	RHESUS	EXPIRY DATE	PACK PUT UP BY			
				TIME	DATE	COMMENTS	SIGNATURE
B147392	A	+	1.10.98				
B147393	A	+	1.10.98				
B147394	A	+	1.10.98				
B147395	A	+	1.10.98				

BLOOD TRANSFUSION   In the event of a reaction stop   Signature...... *A.G.Musker* ....
                        transfusion and notify laboratory   Date........ *29.9.98* ....

14498 GHRJ

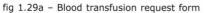

fig 1.29a – Blood transfusion request form

Answers

HEALTH AUTHORITY		24 HOUR INTRAVENOUS FLUID PRESCRIPTION CHART		

DATE   XX – MONTH – YEAR   FOR PATIENTS WITH MORE THAN ONE INTRAVENOUS LINE

CONSULTANT DR LITTLE   WARD FLEMMING   Use computer label if available   Unit No. 123432

HOUSE OFFICER   HOSPITAL ST PETER'S   Surname THOMAS   Forenames DEBRA

Address   Sex M/F

DRUG IDIOSYNCRASY   — NIL —   D of B 13/09/19   Weight

TYPE OF IV FLUID	VOLUME	INFUSION RATE	TIME STARTED	NURSES SIGNATURE	DRUG ADDED AND SOLVENT	DOSE OF DRUG	H O's SIG.	ADDITION TIME	ADDED BY	PHARM

PRESCRIPTION FOR DRUGS TO BE ADDED TO FULL BOTTLE

INTRAVENOUS LINE 1 ; SPECIFY TYPE (eg CVP, Peripheral)   LABEL LINE

DATE Normal Saline	100ml	30Mins								
Blood	1 UNIT	4 Hourly								
Blood	1 UNIT	4 Hourly								
frusemide 40mg (PO) after 2nd unit										
Blood	1 UNIT	4 Hourly								
Blood	1 UNIT	4 Hourly								
Normal Saline	100ml	30mins								
frusemide 40mg (PO) after Normal saline										

Signature

INTRAVENOUS LINE 2 ; SPECIFY TYPE (eg CVP, Peripheral)   LABEL LINE

INTRAVENOUS LINE 3 ; SPECIFY TYPE (eg CVP, Peripheral)   LABEL LINE

INTRAVENOUS FLUID THERAPY SHOULD BE REVIEWED EVERY 24 HOURS AND ALL PREVIOUS REGIMENS CANCELLED
NOTE: THE PRESCRIPTIONS FOR INTRAVENOUS FEEDING MUST BE COMPLETED BY NOON TO ALLOW PHARMACY TO PREPARE THE PRODUCT.

fig 1.29b – Intravenous fluid form

STATION 1.30

Assessment	Good	Adequate	Poor/not done
1 Appropriate introduction (full name and role)	☐	☐	☐
2 Requests the notes and establishes the patient's identity	☐	☐	☐
3 Stops the present unit of blood, checks from the notes the patient and unit details; rechecks the unit and the cross match form	☐	☐	☐
4 Candidate washes their hands using the alcohol handwash provided (no marks if candidate only expresses the need to wash if handwash is provided)	☐	☐	☐
5 Examines the patient to exclude focal signs of sepsis and allergic phenomena (eg wheeze, rashes)	☐	☐	☐
6 Takes blood for:			
Full blood count	☐	☐	☐
Clotting	☐	☐	☐
Re-cross match	☐	☐	☐
Antibody screen	☐	☐	☐
Blood cultures	☐	☐	☐
7 Informs the laboratory that new cross match is required	☐	☐	☐
8 Further sepsis screen: MSU; wound swabs; CXR	☐	☐	☐
9 Asks nursing staff to continue doing observations of temperature, pulse, blood pressure and respiratory rate every 30 minutes for next few hours	☐	☐	☐
10 If transfusion is essential the new unit must be sited as soon as possible	☐	☐	☐

	Good	Adequate	Poor/not done
11 Would explain situation to patient and respond to any concerns	☐	☐	☐
12 Systematic, organised approach	☐	☐	☐

STATION 1.31a

Patient history

I am a 23-year-old bus driver who was admitted for a clot in my right leg, due to being on the pill. No-one has explained the warfarin therapy and I am anxious to learn all about the treatment. I do not have a regular partner and need advice on alternative contraception. I am not allergic to any medications and am not on any regular medicines.

I drink 6 – 8 vodka and tonics on a Saturday night, but cannot drink at other times because of my job. I do not smoke.

I would like to know:

1 How long will I be on the treatment?

2 What happens if I get sick and can't take the tablets?

Assessment	Good	Adequate	Poor/not done
1 Appropriate introduction (full name and role)	☐	☐	☐
2 Explains purpose of interview			
3 Establishes what patient has already been told about treatment	☐	☐	☐
4 Mentions the following points regarding therapy:			
Why patient is taking treatment	☐	☐	☐
Duration of therapy	☐	☐	☐
Importance of compliance	☐	☐	☐
Side-effects principally haemorrhage	☐	☐	☐
What to do in case of haemorrhage	☐	☐	☐

Need for blood monitoring in anticoagulation clinic	☐	☐	☐
Need to carry anticoagulation book	☐	☐	☐
Need for alternative contraception	☐	☐	☐
Interaction with other medications/alcohol	☐	☐	☐
Need to tell dentist or other doctors about treatment	☐	☐	☐
5 Gives clear, jargon-free explanation	☐	☐	☐
6 Checks patient's understanding of information	☐	☐	☐
7 Invites patient's questions and answers appropriately	☐	☐	☐
8 Systematic, organised approach	☐	☐	☐

Answers

Chapter 2: Respiratory Medicine Answers

Chapter 2:

Respiratory Medicine Answers

STATION 2.1

Patient history

I am 23 years old and asthmatic. My asthma is not well controlled. I was first diagnosed aged 14, and have had at least 1 – 2 admissions a year since then. The last admission was three months ago and I was ventilated in intensive care. I have been previously ventilated three times. I continue to smoke 5 – 10 cigarettes a day and have to use my inhalers 3 – 4 times per day. I am at present on salbutamol, Atrovent and Becloforte inhalers and have been on prednisolone 30 mg for the past four days. My normal PEFR when well is 550 l/min.

The present illness started five days ago with a slight head cold but I am now coughing up thick green sputum and am short of breath and wheezy, particularly at night. I am sleeping very badly and feel exhausted, like before I was ventilated the last time. I have had a fever but have not noticed any blood being coughed up or chest pain.

I have no pets and do not know of anything specifically that exacerbates my asthma. I did not have hayfever or eczema as a child and I don't know any other family members who have eczema, asthma or hayfever.

Will I need to be admitted, or will I be able to go home? I feel very upset about this as I'm taking all my medication. Also, I hate being ventilated; being in ITU is really scary.

Assessment	Good	Adequate	Poor/not done
1 Appropriate introduction (full name and role)	☐	☐	☐
2 Explains purpose of interview	☐	☐	☐
3 Establishes duration/initial diagnosis of asthma	☐	☐	☐
4 Establishes normal asthma control, ie medications and the frequency of use; normal PEFR	☐	☐	☐

Answers

5   Establishes previous hospital admissions   ☐   ☐   ☐

6   Establishes if the patient has been
    ventilated in the past   ☐   ☐   ☐

7   Establishes duration and nature
    of the present illness   ☐   ☐   ☐

8   Establishes/excludes the following
    symptoms:

    Cough – nocturnal; daytime   ☐   ☐

    Sputum – volume; colour; consistency   ☐   ☐

    Haemoptysis   ☐   ☐

    Worsening wheeze   ☐   ☐

    Fever   ☐   ☐

    Chest pain – pleuritic   ☐   ☐

    Disturbance of sleep   ☐   ☐

9   Establishes whether patient is a smoker   ☐   ☐   ☐

10 Asks about precipitating factors,
    (eg pets, allergens, occupation)   ☐   ☐   ☐

11 Explains clearly to patient that he
    must be admitted   ☐   ☐   ☐

12 Elicits patient's concerns and responds
    sensitively   ☐   ☐   ☐

13 Appropriate questioning technique   ☐   ☐   ☐

14 Avoids or explains jargon   ☐   ☐   ☐

15 Summarises history back to patient,
    including concerns   ☐   ☐   ☐

16 Systematic, organised approach   ☐   ☐   ☐

SP to Mark

17 The doctors was empathic   ☐   ☐   ☐

Diagnosis
Poorly controlled asthmatic now needing admission due to acute infective
exacerbation

STATION 2.2

Patient history

I am 49 years old and have had a cough for the past 10 days. The cough is generally dry, with occasional clear sputum but no blood. I have been slightly short of breath around the house and have felt dreadful for the past four days, like I've had flu. I have not noticed any wheezing. I have been very feverish in bed at night with drenching sweats. I have not had any other systemic upset. I smoke 20 cigarettes a day and work in the accounts department of a high street bank. I have not been on any foreign travel recently and have not been in contact with anyone else with similar symptoms. I am not on any regular medications and am otherwise well.

Only if asked

I have noticed that two of my prize budgerigars have been very sick recently, in fact one died three days ago.

Assessment	Good	Adequate	Poor/not done
1 Appropriate introduction (full name and role)	☐	☐	☐
2 Explains purpose of interview	☐	☐	☐
3 Establishes duration of presenting complaint	☐	☐	☐
4 Establishes/excludes the following symptoms:			
Cough		☐	☐
Sputum		☐	☐
Haemoptysis		☐	☐
Dyspnoea		☐	☐
Wheeze		☐	☐
Fever		☐	☐
5 Establishes smoking history	☐	☐	☐
6 Establishes risk factors of atypical pneumonia: pets, occupation, foreign travel, contacts	☐	☐	☐
7 Excludes underlying cardiac and respiratory disorders	☐	☐	☐

Answers

	Good	Adequate	Poor/not done
8 Excludes other systemic upset, (eg diarrhoea, confusion, rashes, arthralgia, myalgia)	☐	☐	☐
9 Appropriate questioning technique	☐	☐	☐
10 Avoids or explains jargon	☐	☐	☐
11 Signposts change in focus of questioning	☐	☐	☐
12 Summarises history back to patient	☐	☐	☐
13 Systematic, organised approach	☐	☐	☐
14 Makes a reasonable attempt at diagnosis	☐	☐	☐

Diagnosis

Atypical pneumonia – probably *Chlamydia psittaci*

STATION 2.3

Patient history

I am 61 years old and a retired car factory worker. I am a lifelong smoker, smoking 30 cigarettes a day. I have been getting progressively unwell over the last 2 – 3 years. Every winter for the last 8 – 9 years I have had a severe cough with thick green sputum. This has worsened and now seems to happen all the year round. I can only walk about 50 – 60 metres on the flat without stopping, due to breathlessness and wheeze. I have a near-constant cough and have to sleep with three pillows otherwise I am more breathless. I have never noticed any blood in my sputum and have not been feverish in the past few months. I do not suffer with any chest pains, swelling of the ankles or episodes of breathlessness at night.

My GP recently started me on some inhalers but I rarely use them as they seem to do little good. I take no other regular medications and I am otherwise well, with no other systemic symptoms. I am feeling worried that this is never going to get better. I don't want to become a burden on my wife because she has a lot on her plate. She is the carer for her mother who has dementia.

Assessment	Good	Adequate	Poor/not done
1 Appropriate introduction (full name and role)	☐	☐	☐
2 Explains purpose of interview	☐	☐	☐

3 Establishes duration of presenting
  complaint ☐ ☐ ☐

4 Establishes/excludes the following
  symptoms:

  Cough ☐ ☐

  Sputum ☐ ☐

  Haemoptysis ☐ ☐

  Dyspnoea ☐ ☐

  Wheeze ☐ ☐

  Orthopnoea ☐ ☐

  Exercise tolerance ☐ ☐

  Sleep disturbance ☐ ☐

  Fever ☐ ☐

5 Excludes cardiac symptoms
  (eg angina, oedema) ☐ ☐ ☐

6 Establishes occupational and
  smoking history ☐ ☐ ☐

7 Establishes medication and allergy
  history ☐ ☐ ☐

8 Excludes any other systemic symptoms ☐ ☐ ☐

9 Elicits patient's concerns and responds
  sensitively ☐ ☐ ☐

10 Appropriate questioning technique ☐ ☐ ☐

11 Avoids or explains jargon ☐ ☐ ☐

12 Summarises history back to patient,
   including concerns ☐ ☐ ☐

13 Systematic, organised approach ☐ ☐ ☐

14 Makes a reasonable attempt at
   diagnosis ☐ ☐ ☐

Answers

Diagnosis

Chronic airflow limitation – by definition this patient has chronic bronchitis

STATION 2.4

Patient history

I am 63 years old and a retired plumber. I am a lifelong smoker. I was admitted from the outpatient clinic because of a three month history of weight loss and coughing up blood. Initially the blood was brownish clots mixed in with clear sputum but now there is fresh blood and it occurs 4 – 5 times per day. I have developed a dry irritating cough with breathlessness on exertion. My exercise tolerance is about 500–1000 metres on the flat but I have noticed that I am short of breath at the top of the 14 stairs in my home. I have no history of fever, chest pain, wheeze, difficulty in breathing when lying down or palpitations. I have lost about two stone in weight in the last three months and have felt increasingly lethargic over this time. I do not feel like eating anything at the moment and have no energy or enthusiasm. In the last few weeks my voice has become hoarse.

I have smoked 20 cigarettes a day for the last 35 years, and drink 5 – 10 pints of beer per week. I may have been exposed to asbestos in the past but I'm not sure.

When asked

I am very concerned that I may have cancer and don't want my wife to find out if it is, as I think she would go to pieces. Her father has just died of cancer of the prostate.

Assessment	Good	Adequate	Poor/not done
1 Appropriate introduction (full name and role)	☐	☐	☐
2 Explains purpose of interview	☐	☐	☐
3 Establishes duration of the presenting complaint	☐	☐	☐
4 Characterises the haemoptysis (eg volume, frequency, altered or fresh blood)	☐	☐	☐
5 Establishes associated respiratory symptoms – cough and dyspnoea	☐	☐	☐
6 Excludes other respiratory symptoms – chest pain, sputum and fever	☐	☐	☐
7 Establishes associated symptoms – hoarseness of voice	☐	☐	☐

Answers

8 Establishes systemic symptoms
   of neoplasia – lethargy, malaise,
   loss of weight and appetite ☐ ☐ ☐

9 Establishes smoking and occupational
   history ☐ ☐ ☐

10 Elicits patient's concerns and responds
   sensitively ☐ ☐ ☐

11 Appropriate questioning technique ☐ ☐ ☐

12 Avoids or explains jargon ☐ ☐ ☐

13 Summarises history back to patient,
   including concerns ☐ ☐ ☐

14 Systematic, organised approach ☐ ☐ ☐

15 Makes a reasonable attempt at diagnosis ☐ ☐ ☐

SP to Mark

16 This doctor was easy for me to talk to ☐ ☐ ☐

Diagnosis
Carcinoma of the lung

STATION 2.5

Patient history
I am 18 years old and am normally fit and well. Currently I am studying for my A levels. Last night I developed a sharp pain just under my left breast. The pain has no radiation and has gradually worsened in intensity overnight with no relief from paracetamol. The pain is much worse when I move around, and when I take a deep breath it takes my breath away. I have coughed up two clots of fresh blood this morning but have had no other cough, sputum, or fever. I have become increasingly anxious and breathless over this period.

Risk factors for a pulmonary embolism (only when asked do you admit to these problems).
I recently started on the oral contraceptive pill; I smoke 10 cigarettes a day. My brother died of a clot to the lung suddenly two years ago. I came back on a 23 hour coach journey from Germany two days ago. I am very scared that I am going to die too. I have never had problems with blood clots, thrombosis in my legs, or a clot in my lungs. I have had no injuries recently, and no fractures or operations. I have never been pregnant.

Assessment	Good	Adequate	Poor/not done
1 Appropriate introduction (full name and role)	☐	☐	☐
2 Explains purpose of interview	☐	☐	☐
3 Establishes duration of the symptoms	☐	☐	☐
4 Establishes characteristics of the chest pain – sharp, pleuritic, left midzone, worse on movement, no relief	☐	☐	☐
5 Excludes other respiratory and cardiac symptoms: cough, sputum, wheeze, oedema	☐	☐	☐
6 Establishes history of acute haemoptysis	☐	☐	☐
7 Establishes/excludes risk factors for pulmonary embolism:			
Oral contraceptive pill		☐	☐
Long distance journey		☐	☐
Smoking		☐	☐
Recent major operation		☐	☐
Recent major fracture		☐	☐
Pregnancy		☐	☐
Previous history of PE or DVT		☐	☐
Family history of PE or DVT		☐	☐
History of coagulopathy		☐	☐
8 Establishes no other systemic upset	☐	☐	☐
9 Elicits patient's concerns and responds sensitively	☐	☐	☐
10 Appropriate questioning technique	☐	☐	☐
11 Avoids or explains jargon	☐	☐	☐
12 Summarises history back to patient, including concerns	☐	☐	☐
13 Systematic, organised approach	☐	☐	☐

	Good	Adequate	Poor/not done
14 Establishes the correct diagnosis of pulmonary embolism	☐	☐	☐

SP to Mark

	Good	Adequate	Poor/not done
15 This student was empathic (includes appropriate response to information about brother)	☐	☐	☐

Diagnosis
Left sided pulmonary embolism with multiple risk factors

STATION 2.6

Patient history

I am 16 years old, and I am studying for GCSE exams. Over the last 3 – 4 months I have become increasingly short of breath, particularly when playing sport. The breathlessness initially started during the winter, and was particularly bad when I was playing football in the cold wind. My breathing has slowly worsened and I am now finding it hard to do even short periods of exercise.

I have been sleeping badly because of a persistent cough and wheezing during the night, and I am now having to sleep with three pillows. I have not had any sputum, fever, coughing up of blood or swelling of my ankles.

I smoke 2 – 3 cigarettes at weekends but recently have had to stop because it makes me very wheezy. I have some goldfish but no other pets, and have never had eczema, hayfever or asthma. My brother and my mother both have eczema and my sister has asthma. I'm worried that I'm getting asthma too. I'm also very concerned whether this is all going to affect my studying.

Assessment	Good	Adequate	Poor/not done
1 Appropriate introduction (full name and role)	☐	☐	☐
2 Explains purpose of interview	☐	☐	☐
3 Establishes duration of present illness	☐	☐	☐
4 Establishes exacerbating factors of breathlessness	☐	☐	☐
5 Establishes associated symptoms – nocturnal cough, wheeze, orthopnoea	☐	☐	☐

6 Excludes other respiratory symptoms –
   sputum, haemoptysis, fever and chest
   pain

7 Establishes lack of sleep due to cough
   and wheeze

8 Establishes/excludes associated
   risk factors – smoking, pets, pollen
   and dust

9 Establishes history of atopy

10 Establishes family history of
   asthma and atopy

11 Elicits patient's concerns and responds
   sensitively

12 Appropriate questioning technique

13 Avoids or explains jargon

14 Summarises history back to patient,
   including concerns

15 Systematic, organised approach

SP to Mark

16 Makes a reasonable attempt at
   the diagnosis

Diagnosis
New onset of asthma

STATION 2.7

Assessment	Good	Adequate	Poor/not done
1 Appropriate introduction (full name and role)	☐	☐	☐
2 Gains verbal consent – explains examination to patient	☐	☐	☐
3 Candidate washes their hands using the alcohol handwash provided (no marks if candidate only expresses the need to wash if handwash is provided)	☐	☐	☐
4 Stands at the end of the bed and comments on wellbeing of patient. Times and comments on the respiratory rate	☐	☐	☐
5 Comments on the presence/absence of – peripheral oedema; abdominal breathing; use of accessory muscles; intercostals recession; tracheal tug; peripheral/central cyanosis/anaemia; pectus excavatum/carinatum; skeletal deformity; plethora; cushingoid appearance.	☐	☐	☐
6 Comments on presence/absence of O_2 via mask or nasal cannulae/sputum pot; nebuliser; PEFR chart; O_2 saturation chart; inhalers	☐	☐	☐
7 Returns to patient's right hand side to examine the hands. Comments on presence/absence of:			
Clubbing		☐	☐
Anaemia		☐	☐
'CO$_2$ peripheries' – warm venodilated/ bounding pulse	☐	☐	☐
Peripheral cyanosis		☐	☐
Tar staining		☐	☐

Answers

If appropriate mentions need to assess for asterixis ☐ ☐

8 Examines the face commenting on presence/absence of anaemia, plethora and central cyanosis ☐ ☐ ☐

9 Examines the trachea – commenting on position ☐ ☐ ☐

10 Attempts to examine for lymphadenopathy ☐ ☐

(**Examiner to stop student**)

11 Re-examines and comments on presence/absence of thoracotomy scars, aspiration sites and old chest drain scars. ☐ ☐ ☐

12 Examines for **and** correctly demonstrates expansion of the chest (anterior) ☐ ☐ ☐

13 Percusses the anterior chest using:

Correct technique ☐ ☐ ☐

Comparison of two sides ☐ ☐ ☐

Anatomical/clinically correct positions ☐ ☐ ☐

14 Auscultates the anterior chest:

Comparing the two sides ☐ ☐

Listens in clinically correct positions ☐ ☐

15 Examines for vocal or tactile vocal fremitus:

Using correct technique ☐ ☐

Comparing two sides ☐ ☐

16 Percusses, auscultates and examines in the right axilla for right middle lobe pathology ☐ ☐ ☐

17 Examines **and** correctly demonstrates expansion of posterior chest ☐ ☐ ☐

18 Percusses the posterior chest using:

Correct technique ☐ ☐

Comparison of two sides ☐ ☐

Clinically correct positions ☐ ☐

19 Auscultates the posterior chest:

Compares the two sides ☐ ☐

Listens in clinically correct positions ☐ ☐

20 Examines for vocal or tactile vocal fremitus:

Using correct technique ☐ ☐ ☐

Comparing the two sides ☐ ☐ ☐

21 Repositions patient – ensuring comfort
and dignity; thanks patient ☐ ☐ ☐

22 Completes examination by asking for
PEFR reading; O_2 saturation; temperature
and to see contents of sputum pot
(if available) ☐ ☐ ☐

23 Presents findings in a fluent, logical
manner ☐ ☐ ☐

24 Presents an appropriate differential
diagnosis or causes and complications ☐ ☐ ☐

Answers

STATION 2.8

Assessment	Good	Adequate	Poor/not done
1 Appropriate introduction (full name and role)	☐	☐	☐
2 Explains examination and gains verbal consent	☐	☐	☐
3 Candidate washes their hands using the alcohol handwash provided (no marks if candidate only expresses the need to wash if handwash is provided)	☐	☐	☐
4 Stands at the end of the bed and comments on presence/absence of: patient distress; tachypnoea; brachypnoea; peripheral oedema; abdominal breathing; use of accessory muscles; intercostals recession; tracheal tug; peripheral/central cyanosis/anaemia; pectus excavatum/carinatum; skeletal deformity; plethora; cushingoid appearance	☐	☐	☐
5 Comments on presence/ absence of O_2/sputum pot; nebuliser; PEFR chart; O_2 saturation; inhalers	☐	☐	☐
6 Examines the trachea commenting on position	☐	☐	☐
7 Offers to examine cervical, supraclavicular and axillary lymphadenopathy	☐	☐	☐

(**Examiner to stop student**)

	Good	Adequate	Poor/not done
8 Re-examines and comments on presence/ absence of thoracotomy scars, aspiration sites and old chest drain scars.	☐	☐	☐
9 Examines for **and** correctly demonstrates expansion of the chest (anterior)	☐	☐	☐

10 Percusses the anterior chest using:

   Correct technique ☐ ☐

   Comparison of two sides ☐ ☐

   Anatomical/clinically correct positions ☐ ☐

11 Auscultates the anterior chest:

   Comparing the two sides ☐ ☐

   Listens in clinically correct positions ☐ ☐

12 Examines for vocal or tactile vocal fremitus:

   Using correct technique ☐ ☐

   Comparing two sides ☐ ☐

13 Percusses, auscultates and examines
   in the right axilla for right middle
   lobe pathology ☐ ☐ ☐

14 Repositions patient – ensuring comfort
   and dignity; thanks patient ☐ ☐ ☐

15 Completes examination by asking for
   PEFR reading; O_2 saturation; temperature
   and to see contents of sputum pot
   (if available) ☐ ☐ ☐

16 Presents findings in a fluent, logical
   manner. ☐ ☐ ☐

17 Presents an appropriate differential
   diagnosis or causes and complications ☐ ☐ ☐

Answers

STATION 2.9

Assessment	Good	Adequate	Poor/not done
1 Appropriate introduction (full name and role)	☐	☐	☐
2 Explains examination and gains verbal consent	☐	☐	☐
3 Candidate washes their hands using the alcohol handwash provided (no marks if candidate only expresses the need to wash if handwash is provided)	☐	☐	☐
4 Stands at the end of the bed and comments on presence/absence of – patient distress; tachypnoea; brachypnoea; peripheral oedema; abdominal breathing; use of accessory muscles; intercostals recession; tracheal tug; peripheral/central cyanosis/anaemia; pectus excavatum/ carinatum; skeletal deformity; plethora; cyanosis	☐	☐	☐
5 Comments on presence/absence of O_2/ sputumpot; nebuliser; PEFR chart; O_2 saturation chart; inhalers	☐	☐	☐
6 Examines for and comments on presence/absence of thoracotomy scars and aspiration sites	☐	☐	☐
7 Examines for and demonstrates correctly expansion of the posterior chest	☐	☐	☐
8 Percusses the posterior chest using:			
Correct technique		☐	☐
Comparison of two sides		☐	☐
Clinically correct positions		☐	☐
9 Auscultates the posterior chest			
Compares the two sides		☐	☐
Listens in clinically correct positions		☐	☐

10 Examines for vocal or tactile vocal fremitus:

Using correct technique ☐ ☐

Comparing the two sides ☐ ☐

11 Repositions patient – ensuring comfort
and dignity; thanks patient ☐ ☐ ☐

12 Completes examination by asking for
PEFR reading; O_2 saturation; temperature
and to see contents of sputum pot
(if available) ☐ ☐ ☐

13 Presents findings in a fluent, logical
manner ☐ ☐ ☐

14 Presents an appropriate differential
diagnosis or causes and presence/absence
of complications ☐ ☐ ☐

Common pathologies which should be considered when asked to examine the:

1 Anterior chest

(a) Apical fibrosis: Old TB; extrinsic allergic bronchioloalveolitis (EABA); ankylosing spondylitis; pancoast tumours; pneumoconioses, radiotherapy (COMMON in OSCEs)

(b) Large pleural effusions – transudates/ exudates

(c) COPD or asthma (COMMON in OSCEs)

(d) Old TB – apical fibrosis, plombage, thoracoplasty

(e) Old lobectomy or pneumonectomy (scars will be posterior therefore unseen from the anterior examination (if not looked for!))

(f) Pancoast tumour: look for an ipsilateral Horner's syndrome; wasting in TI distribution (1st interosseal space), pleural effusion

2 Posterior chest

(a) Basal fibrosis: idiopathic pulmonary fibrosis; fibrosis 2° to rheumatoid disease or asbestosis (COMMON in OSCEs)

(b) Pleural effusions – transudates/exudates (less common in OSCEs)

(c) COPD – reduced breath sounds at base (COMMON in OSCEs)

Answers

STATION 2.10

Assessment	Good	Adequate	Poor/not done
1 Appropriate introduction (full name and role)	☐	☐	☐
2 Explains the procedure and gains verbal consent	☐	☐	☐
3 Explains/ demonstrates how to perform peak flow mentioning/ demonstrating the following:			
Returning gauge to zero		☐	☐
Holding meter with fingers away from gauge		☐	☐
Takes as big an inspiration as possible		☐	☐
Places mouthpiece into mouth with lips sealed around it		☐	☐
Blows out 'as quickly as possible'		☐	☐
Peak flow meter records the rate, ie 'how quickly' – NOT how long or how much the you blow out		☐	☐
Peak flow should be performed standing up where possible		☐	☐
4 Allows patient three attempts following and correcting patient's technique	☐	☐	☐
5 Correctly explains 'best of three' result using the tables provided	☐	☐	☐
6 Invites questions and answers appropriately	☐	☐	☐
7 Thanks patient and brings consultation to a formal conclusion	☐	☐	☐

You should know factors which influence PEFR including height, age, sex, acute and chronic respiratory disease, smoking.

This station is often used in conjunction with demonstration/checking inhaler technique.

STATION 2.11

1 (E) (c)

This man has chronic respiratory failure causing pulmonary hypertension, right sided heart failure and polycythaemia. Management may include regular venesection with an aim to reduce the haematocrit (Hct) to less than 0.50.

2 (C) (d)

The patient has a microcytic anaemia secondary to gastrointestinal blood loss due to her NSAID treatment. Chronic rheumatoid arthritis may also cause a microcytic anaemia through the anaemia of chronic disease.

3 (A) (b)

This patient is suffering from a grossly raised platelet count or thrombocytosis. This is an uncommon cause of thromboembolic disease leading to deep vein thrombosis (DVT) and myocardial infarction, CVAs and limb ischaemia.

4 (B) (e)

Mycoplasma pneumonia causes several haematological problems including haemolytic anaemia, a depressed white cell count with a relative lymphopenia and thrombocytopenia. The haemolysis is confirmed by the reticulocytosis causing the raised MCV.

5 (D) (a)

Sickle cell disease is one of the most common haemoglobinopathies, being particularly prevalent amongst Afrocaribbean races. It often presents as an acute sickle crisis due to infection, drugs or metabolic disturbance. Acute sickle crises are characterised by bony pain, pneumonitis, splenic pain and infarction, and acute haemolysis.

Answers

STATION 2.12

1 (C) (e)

The carcinoid syndrome is more commonly associated with gastrointestinal tumours but is well recognised with pulmonary lesions. The tumours produce 5HT which is responsible for the wheeze and diarrhoea. The flushing is caused by various mediators including substance P, kallikrein and bradykinins.

2 (D) (c)

Hypercalcaemia associated with lung tumours may be caused by ectopic parathormone, bony metastases, cyclic-AMP-stimulating factor or a prostaglandin. Ectopic parathormone is most commonly expressed by squamous cell carcinoma. Initial therapy should include intravenousrehydration and hydrocortisone but the use of intravenous bisphosphonates, followed by oral maintenance therapy, has now become the standard treatment.

3 (E) (d)

The SIADH in this case may be caused by a primary lung tumour or cerebral metastases. Both may be responsible for these symptoms and, after correction of the hyponatraemia, a CT head scan should be performed. SIADH is proven by a paired urinary and plasma osmolality, where the urinary osmolality is raised relative to the plasma osmolality. The urinary sodium may be normal or raised but the plasma sodium is always low. Other criteria for diagnosing SIADH include normal renal and adrenal function and the absence of hypotension, hypovolaemia and oedema.

4 (B) (a)

Lung tumours metastasise to cervical, supraclavicular and contralateral hilar lymph nodes, the brain, liver and bone. The enlarged liver feels hard and 'craggy' and may present with jaundice or deranged LFTs.

5 (A) (b)

Small cell tumours and bronchial carcinoid may both produce ectopic ACTH. The patient presents with the familiar clinical features of Cushing's syndrome but is characterised by severe malaise and hypokalaemic alkalosis. Metyrapone and, more rarely, ketoconazole, are used to block the synthesis of cortisol but tumour excision remains the best treatment.

STATION 2.13

1 (F) (g)
Sarcoidosis is now thought to be due to an, as yet undefined, allergen causing an abnormal T helper cell response. It causes bilateral hilar lymphadenopathy and mid and upper zone pulmonary fibrosis.

2 (E) (f)
Wegener's granulomatosis is made up of a classical triad of upper and lower respiratory tract symptoms and renal failure. The disease is characterised by the presence of the cANCA antibody, in particular the antiproteinase 3 antibody, which is directly involved in the pathogenesis of the disorder.

3 (B) (a)
Churg-Strauss is a variant of polyarteritis nodosa (PAN). It presents in young adults with asthma, peripheral eosinophilia, subcutaneous lesions, peripheral neuropathy and vasculitis. Unlike PAN it rarely involves the kidneys. The non-specific pANCA (anti-myeloperoxidase antibody), has been identified in this disorder but cannot be used to characterise it, as it is found in many other immune based diseases including inflammatory bowel disease and autoimmune hepatitis.

4 (C) (e)
Goodpasture's syndrome is the association of pulmonary haemorrhage and an acute glomerulonephritis. It has now been renamed antiglomerular basement membrane disease. The autoantibody is directed against type IV collagen, which is common to the basement membrane in both the glomeruli and the alveoli.

5 (G) (c)
Rheumatoid arthritis commonly affects the lungs. The principal respiratory presentations include pleurisy and exudative pleural effusions. Pulmonary fibrosis, similar to cryptogenic fibrosing alveolitis, pulmonary nodules and 'honeycombing', may also occur.

6 (A) (d)
Systemic lupus erythematosus does not affect the lungs as commonly as rheumatoid arthritis. It may produce an exudative effusion and rarely pulmonary fibrosis.

7 (D) (b)
Progressive systemic sclerosis is characterised by the antiSCL – 70 antibody. The lungs are commonly affected by fibrosis which may become generalised with 'honeycombing' and pulmonary hypertension.

Answers

STATION 2.14

1 (D) (c)

This patient has Guillain-Barré syndrome with both motor and sensory neuropathy, the blood gas results infer type II respiratory failure, the pH is normal. The HCO_3^- is normal which shows this patient does not normally retain CO_2. The patient is young and this set of blood gases infer he is tiring with poor respiratory effort, a similar picture may be found in severe asthma. The treatment of choice is ventilation and plasmapheresis.

2 (E) (d)

This man has acute pulmonary oedema which causes a type I respiratory failure. He also has a metabolic acidosis shown by the low pH and HCO_3^-, this is probably due to a lactic acidosis caused by poor tissue oxygenation.

3 (B) (e)

These results are consistent with type II respiratory failure, a respiratory acidosis and compensatory metabolic alkalosis. This combination is seen in chronic CO_2 retainers where the respiratory acidosis is caused by the retention of CO_2 and the metabolic alkalosis by the retention of HCO_3^-. These patients should be given 24% (28% maximum) O_2 therapy.

4 (C) (a)

This patient has had a PE and demonstrates type I respiratory failure with a respiratory alkalosis. She is hypoxic which is important to note as occasionally such patients are diagnosed as 'hysterical' and are given a paper bag to rebreathe into! Type I failure in this age group is always pathological and should be taken seriously.

5 (A) (b)

This patient has a respiratory alkalosis but has no respiratory failure. She has been hyperventilating and this is shown by the supersaturated high levels of oxygen with low CO_2. This patient should be treated with a rebreathing bag and reassurance.

STATION 2.15

1 A	6 C
2 B and C	7 B
3 A +/– B	8 A
4 B and C	9 A, B and C
5 B	10 A and C

Comment

Patient (A) – demonstrates a restrictive lung defect with resting hypoxia and reduced transfer coefficient. In view of the history of rheumatoid arthritis this picture would fit with fibrosing alveolitis. These patients have type I respiratory failure and classically the hypoxia worsens with exercise.

Patient (B) – the history and lung function tests suggest underlying obstructive airways disease. The reduced transfer coefficient suggests probable emphysema and excludes late onset asthma. The data do not indicate whether there is any reversibility. This is demonstrated by repeating the FEV1 and FVC tests pre- and postnebuliser. Demonstration of reversibility is important as it indicates whether inhaled steroid therapy may be useful.

Patient (C) – this history is suggestive of myasthenia gravis. These patients get an obstructive lung defect as they are unable to move their chest wall due to the neuromuscular defect. The transfer coefficient is normal as there is no alveolar problem.

Answers

STATION 2.16

(A) Trachea

(B) Right 5th rib (anterior aspect)

(C) Left 7th rib (posterior aspect)

(D) Aortic knuckle

(E) Left heart border (left ventricle)

(F) Right pulmonary artery

(G) Right costodiaphragmatic angle

(H) Gastric air bubble

(I) Right heart border (right atrium)

(J) ECG sticker

1 **True**	6 **True**
2 **True**	7 **True**
3 **False**	8 **False**
4 **False**	9 **False**
5 **False**	10 **False**

This is a well-centred PA chest radiograph of an elderly woman. The cardiothoracic ratio is normal. There is calcification within the aortic knuckle probably due to atherosclerotic degeneration. There is no evidence of soft tissue abnormalities, cardiac failure, perforated viscus or fractures. The bones are relatively osteopenic but there is little evidence of arthritic degeneration. There are eight anterior ribs visible and flattening of the diaphragm which indicates a degree of hyperexpansion.

STATION 2.17

(a) 1 True 2 False 3 False 4 True 5 True
This is a PA poorly penetrated CXR showing hyperexpanded lung fields and flattened diaphragms. There is marked pulmonary apical fibrosis resulting in the hilar being pulled upwards towards the apices. The fibrosis was secondary to tuberculosis in this patient, other causes include pneumoconiosis, ankylosing spondylitis, rheumatoid arthritis and malignancy.

(b) 1 False 2 False 3 True 4 True 5 False
This is a well-penetrated, well-centred PA chest radiograph showing a cavitating area in the left apex. The commonest cause of this appearance is tuberculosis. Other causes of cavitation include *Staphylococcus*, *Klebsiella*, *Pseudomonas*, fungal infection and malignancy.

(c) 1 True 2 False 3 False 4 False 5 False
This is a well-penetrated, slightly rotated chest radiograph showing a right middle lobe pneumonia, with loss of definition of the right heart border. A lateral view would show the consolidated lobe. The heart and left lung are normal.

(d) 1 True 2 True 3 True 4 True 5 False
This is quite a complicated radiograph to interpret correctly. There is loss of the right costodiaphragmatic angle, with multiple fluid levels above it. There is a 10%, by area, pneumothorax clearly seen in the right upper/mid zone. There is also blunting of the left costodiaphragmatic angle. This represents a right hydropneumothorax with adhesions causing the fluid levels and a small left pleural effusion. This patient had tuberculosis. Causes of pleural effusions should be divided by their protein content, into transudates (< 30g/l) and exudates (> 30g/l).

(e) 1 True 2 False 3 False 4 True 5 False
This is an AP chest radiograph showing a near 100% by area right sided pneumothorax. There is a chest drain in situ (just), with a kink seen at the skin entry site, possibly explaining why there has been no re-expansion of the lung. When describing a pneumothorax one should describe the size, by the area of the lung field occupied by the air within the hemithorax. The costodiaphragmatic angles have been missed on this radiograph and a repeat film should be requested to comment fully on the chest.

(f) 1 True 2 False 3 True 4 True 5 False
This a well-centred PA chest radiograph showing a large round mass in the right mid/lower zone. The most likely cause of this appearance is a bronchogenic carcinoma; this was confirmed on sputum cytology. The lung fields are hyperexpanded with flattened hemidiaphragms indicating probable chronic airways disease, most likely caused by cigarette smoking. There are no bone metastases seen.

STATION 2.18

(a) 1 False 2 False 3 False 4 True 5 False

This is a poorly penetrated PA chest radiograph showing multiple round lesions in both lung fields. These are consistent with 'cannonball' metastases, which commonly arise from breast, testicular, thyroid, renal or gastrointestinal primaries and in malignant trophoblastic disease. In children they may arise from Ewing's sarcoma and osteogenic sarcoma. Multiple round lesions may also be produced by infections, eg abscesses, coccidioidomycosis, histoplasmosis and hydatid disease, Wegener's and Caplan's syndrome.

(b) 1 True 2 False 3 True 4 False 5 True

This is a PA chest radiograph showing bilateral hilar lymphadenopathy (BHL). The differential diagnosis includes sarcoidosis, lymphoma, tuberculosis and bronchial carcinoma. The bones are normal and there is no evidence of myeloma.

(c) 1 True 2 False 3 True 4 False 5 True

This radiograph shows evidence of peribronchial thickening and basal cystic changes consistent with bronchiectasis. This may be caused by childhood infections, eg whooping cough and measles, aspiration of a foreign body and proximal obstruction due to mucus plugging or hilar masses, eg tuberculosis or malignancy. The commonest inherited cause is cystic fibrosis; other rare disorders include Kartagener's syndrome, Williams-Campbell syndrome and immunodeficiencies such as hypogammaglobulinaemia and Chédiak-Higashi syndrome.

(d) 1 False 2 False 3 True 4 False 5 True

This radiograph shows evidence of collapse/consolidation of the right upper lobe. The horizontal fissure is elevated due to loss of volume. Lobar collapse is principally caused by proximal obstruction of the bronchus. In this case there was a central obstructing carcinoma.

(e) 1 False 2 False 3 False 4 True 5 True

This radiograph shows a retrocardiac shadow causing a 'double' left heart border. This is due to left lower collapse which may be easily overlooked.

STATION 2.19

(a)

(A) Trachea

(B) Sternum

(C) Left sternoclavicular joint

(D) Thoracic vertebra

(E) Ribs

(F) Right scapula

(G) Left lung

(H) SVC

(I) Oesophagus

(b)

(A) Left main bronchus

(B) Oesophagus

(C) Right main bronchus

(D) Descending thoracic aorta

(E) Termination of the SVC

(F) Right scapula

(G) Thoracic vertebra (T6)

(H) Ascending thoracic aorta

(I) Pulmonary trunk division

Answers

STATION 2.20

1 This is an AP chest radograph showing a grossly enlarged aortic knuckle, consistent with a thoracic aortic aneurysm. There is evidence of calcification about 1 cm from the edge of the dilated area suggesting dissection away from the true wall of the aorta, (marked by the calcification).

2 The CT scan of the thorax confirms the presence of a dissecting thoracic aortic aneurysm. The structures labelled are:

(A) Sternum

(B) Ascending thoracic aorta

(C) Trachea

(D) Dissecting aneurysm of the descending thoracic aorta

(E) Superior vena cava

3 This is a venogram of the left lower limb showing a filling defect in the superficial femoral and calf veins. This is consistent with a DVT and requires anticoagulation. With the introduction of low molecular weight/fractionated heparins, patients can now receive a standard, once-daily subcutaneous heparin injection, the dose being calculated by their weight. Patients with proven DVT should be anticoagulated with heparin and then started on warfarin for at least three months. Underlying risk factors such as the use of the OCP should be removed, and patients with no obvious cause investigated for possible coagulopathies. A coagulopathy screen should be performed prior to anticoagulation and should include: INR, APPT, Factor V Leiden, anticardiolipin antibody and proteins C and S levels. Venography is relatively expensive and technically difficult in a swollen limb; it is being superseded by colour Doppler ultrasound of the veins.

STATION 2.21

(a) This is a radiolabelled ventilation (V)/perfusion (Q) scan showing a mismatched defect in the right lower lobe. The patient is asked to inhale a radiolabelled gas and is then injected with a contrast medium. Three outcomes are possible.

1 A normal scan – all areas are ventilated and perfused

2 Matched defects – areas of the lungs have both poor ventilation and perfusion. This arises in patients with pre-existing lung disease, eg fibrosis, bronchiectasis and chronic airways disease. V/Q scans in such patients are often difficult to interpret and other modes of investigation should be employed.

3 Mismatched defects – as in the scan shown there are areas of normal ventilation with poor/no perfusion. This implies pulmonary embolism.

4 Patients with mismatched defects should be formally anticoagulated with heparin (this should have already been started) and then warfarin. They should receive warfarin for at least six months and any underlying risk factors, such as being on the OCP, should be addressed.

(b) This patient has had pulmonary angiography showing a massive pulmonary embolism cutting off the blood supply to the right lower lobe and most of the left lung. This represents a 'saddle' embolism which sits across the pulmonary arteries. The longer of the two radio-opaque tubes represents the Swan-Gantz catheter through which the contrast medium has been delivered. The other more centrally located tube is an endotracheal tube. Treatment of such massive emboli is still extremely difficult and the prognosis remains very poor. One treatment which has been tried is violent thrusting of the Swan-Gantz catheter in and out of the pulmonary artery while injecting streptokinase through it. Surgical evacuation of the embolus under extracorporeal circulatory bypass is successful in selected patients.

STATION 2.22

Patient history

I am 22 years old and have been recently diagnosed as asthmatic. I am unemployed at present but am hoping to get a job in retailing. I was meant to see the respiratory specialist nurse yesterday about how to use my inhalers but she was away sick. I have very little idea of how to use them but have watched the other patients on the ward using theirs. I am a non-smoker. I am not very good at understanding exactly what doctors tell me so I would like a very clear and simple explanation. I would like to know whether I should use the inhaler before vigorous exercise like sex.

Assessment	Good	Adequate	Poor/not done
1 Appropriate introduction (full name and role)	☐	☐	☐
2 Explains what interview is to be about	☐	☐	☐
3 Establishes patient's present understanding of the treatment	☐	☐	☐
4 Explains use of the inhaler, covering the following points:			
(1) Shake the inhaler with the cap on		☐	☐
(2) Remove the cap from the mouthpiece		☐	☐
(3) Take breath in and then fully exhale		☐	☐
(4) Place mouthpiece into mouth		☐	☐
(5) Synchronously take a deep breath in as you press the top of the inhaler down		☐	☐
(6) Repeat from step (3) to step (5)		☐	☐
5 Explains about gargling/rinsing out mouth after using steroid inhaler	☐	☐	☐
6 Establishes patient understanding allowing him to demonstrate technique	☐	☐	☐
7 Explains to patient correct situations to use inhalers, ie prophylactic and regular use	☐	☐	☐
8 Gives clear, jargon-free explanation	☐	☐	☐

Assessment	Good	Adequate	Poor/not done
9 Invites patient to ask questions, and answers appropriately	☐	☐	☐
10 Systematic, organised approach	☐	☐	☐

STATION 2.23

Patient history

I am 31 years old and I have asthma, which is not well controlled. I have been ventilated twice in the last year and the consultant has decided that I need to be put on steroids for the foreseeable future. I am very anxious, as I have heard that steroids can make you very fat and give you terrible acne. I am reluctant to take the tablets and since discharge from the hospital I have missed several doses. I am also worried about my diabetes which, up till now, has been quite well controlled.

Assessment	Good	Adequate	Poor/not done
1 Appropriate introduction (full name and role)	☐	☐	☐
2 Explains purpose of interview	☐	☐	☐
3 Establishes patient's understanding and anxieties about steroid therapy	☐	☐	☐
4 Explains the need for the addition of the steroids	☐	☐	☐
5 Explains the following about the steroid therapy:			
Must never miss a dose	☐	☐	☐
If too sick to take the tablets, should seek medical help	☐	☐	☐
Check patient has a steroid card	☐	☐	☐
6 Explains long-term side-effects of the steroids:			
Thinning and bruising of the skin	☐	☐	☐
Cushing's and Addison's syndromes	☐	☐	☐
Hypertension	☐	☐	☐
Acne and weight gain (reversible)	☐	☐	☐

	Good	Adequate	Poor/not done
7 Explains the effects on diabetes and the need to closely monitor control. Probable need to increase insulin	☐	☐	☐
8 Gives clear, jargon-free explanation	☐	☐	☐
9 Checks patient's understanding of information	☐	☐	☐
10 Invites patient questions, and answers appropriately	☐	☐	☐
11 Systematic, organised approach	☐	☐	☐

STATION 2.24

Patient history

I am 64 years old and have been diagnosed with chronic airways limitation. I have had several admissions to hospital in the last year with chest problems and nearly died on this admission. The doctors want to put me on oxygen treatment at home but I am not very keen. I have just given up smoking in the last three months but occasionally sneak a puff from my husband, who continues to smoke. I don't think he will give it up for anything! I do not think any new treatment will help me, and I am resigned to dying in the next few months. However, now you have told me the oxygen may help my illness and actually decrease my likelihood of dying I should like to give it a chance.

Assessment	Good	Adequate	Poor/not done
1 Appropriate introduction (full name and role)	☐	☐	☐
2 Explains what interview will be about	☐	☐	☐
3 Explores patient's understanding of the oxygen therapy and her anxieties about the treatment	☐	☐	☐
4 Ensures patient has stopped smoking and understands the dangers of smoking around oxygen	☐	☐	☐

5 Explains wearing oxygen for over 15 hours
  per day will decrease periods of illness
  and, over longer periods (19+ hours
  per day), may increase life expectancy ☐ ☐ ☐

6 Offers to explain about oxygen to
  patient's husband ☐ ☐ ☐

7 Gives clear, jargon-free explanation ☐ ☐ ☐

8 Invites patient questions and answers
  appropriately ☐ ☐ ☐

9 Systematic, organised approach ☐ ☐ ☐

SP to Mark

10 The doctor was empathic ☐ ☐ ☐

Answers

Comment

To qualify for home oxygen therapy a patient must have a resting $PaO_2 < 7.3$ kPa; $PaCO_2 > 6.0$ kPa; FEV1 < 1.5 litres, FVC < 2.0 litres. They must have stopped smoking and the dangers of smoking with oxygen therapy must be explained clearly. Studies have shown that maintaining these patients on oxygen for 15+ hours a day decreases their morbidity and for 19+ hours a day decreases their mortality. Two oxygen points are set up around the house, usually in the sitting room and the bedroom. Patients do not have to pay for their therapy, which is often a major concern. The oxygen must be prescribed by their GP and must, therefore, be agreed with them before therapy can be instituted.

STATION 2.25a

Patient history

I am 53 years old and have come to the day-care centre for a bronchoscopy. I have been told by the registrar in the outpatient clinic that I have a 'shadow' on the chest X-ray, which needs to be looked at. I am unsure about the procedure and am quite anxious about it. I have been told a camera is passed into the lung but I am very confused by this.

I am anxious to have as much information as possible, both about the tests and about what might be wrong.

At the end of the consultation you should ask the doctor – 'Do you think that the shadow on the chest X-ray is cancer?'

Assessment	Good	Adequate	Poor/not done
1 Appropriate introduction (full name and role)	☐	☐	☐
2 Establishes identity of patient and reason for attendance	☐	☐	☐
3 Establishes present understanding of the procedure	☐	☐	☐
4 Explains the common complications post procedure:			
Sore throat		☐	☐
Drowsiness		☐	☐
Chest discomfort		☐	☐
5 Explains the uncommon complications of the procedure:			
Surgical emphysema		☐	☐
Pneumothorax		☐	☐
Pneumomediastinum		☐	☐
6 Gives clear, jargon-free explanation	☐	☐	☐
7 Checks patient's understanding of information	☐	☐	☐

8 Invites questions and answers
   appropriately   ☐   ☐   ☐

9 Systematic, organised approach   ☐   ☐   ☐

10   Deals with the issue of the mass on
   the CXR in a sympathetic, sensitive
   manner   ☐   ☐   ☐

SP to Mark

11 This doctor was empathetic   ☐   ☐   ☐

Answers

Chapter 3: Rheumatology and Dermatology Answers

Chapter 3

Rheumatology and Dermatology Answers

STATION 3.1

Patient history

I am a 23-year-old woman and work in IT as a programme developer. I was fit and well until three months ago. Initially I had joint pains, particularly in my fingers and toes, but more recently I have had swelling and severe pain in the small joints of my hands. The arthritis affects both hands identically and is associated with feeling generally unwell, tiredness and fever. I have also had painful, red eyes and chest pain with when I breathe in, over the past few weeks. I have not had any large joint swelling or pain, and no back pain. I am generally otherwise well and have had no bowel or urogenital symptoms. I am on the oral contraceptive pill but no other medications. I do not know anyone else in my family who has had arthritis. I am upset because it has taken weeks to get this appointment and I am now finding it hard to use a keyboard.

Assessment	Good	Adequate	Poor/not done
1 Appropriate introduction (full name and role)	☐	☐	☐
2 Explains purpose of the interview	☐	☐	☐
3 Establishes the presenting complaint and duration of symptoms	☐	☐	☐
4 Establishes the characteristics of the arthritis: *Symmetrical versus asymmetrical involvement*	☐	☐	☐
Small joint involvement – proximal or distal	☐	☐	☐
Large joints involved – upper and lower limbs	☐	☐	☐

Spine – cervical, thoracic,
lumbar, sacroiliac ☐ ☐ ☐

Features of acute arthritis – swelling,
pain, increased temperature, erythema ☐ ☐ ☐

Early morning stiffness ☐ ☐ ☐

5 Establishes/excludes systemic
associations:
Eye/visual problems ☐ ☐ ☐

Bowel – upper/lower GI symptoms ☐ ☐ ☐

Respiratory symptoms ☐ ☐ ☐

Urogenital symptoms ☐ ☐ ☐

Skin, nail and hair problems ☐ ☐ ☐

General systemic symptoms –
fever, malaise, arthralgia, myalgia ☐ ☐ ☐

6 Establishes/excludes family
history of arthritis ☐ ☐ ☐

7 Establishes medication history ☐ ☐ ☐

8 Establishes previous medical history –
particularly autoimmune disease ☐ ☐ ☐

9 Elicits patient's concerns and responds
sensitively ☐ ☐ ☐

10 Appropriate questioning technique ☐ ☐ ☐

11 Avoids or explains jargon ☐ ☐ ☐

12 Summarises history back to patient,
including concerns ☐ ☐ ☐

13 Makes a reasonable attempt at the
diagnosis ☐ ☐ ☐

14 Systematic, organised approach ☐ ☐ ☐

SP to Mark

15 I found this student empathic ☐ ☐ ☐

Diagnosis
Acute rheumatoid arthritis with episcleritis and pleuritic chest pain

STATION 3.2

Patient history

I am 16 years old and still at school. I was fit and well until about three or four months ago, started to get lower back pain. Initially I put it down to increased rugby training. The pain is in my lower back and upper buttocks and radiates down the upper thighs to my knee. It is a dull ache, which is much worse in the mornings, and is associated with stiffness, particularly on getting out of bed and after sitting on the 45 minute bus ride to school. The pain has been eased by aspirin tablets and I find that the stiffness eases through the day. I have noticed more recently that my neck is also starting to feel stiff. There are no other joints involved and I have been otherwise well. I have had no eye, breathing, bowel or urinary symptoms.

I have only previously been in hospital once, for a tonsillectomy. I am on no other medications other than the aspirin and do not drink any alcohol or smoke cigarettes. My mother has psoriasis and my grandfather had severe back pain associated with his Crohn's disease.

This is really starting to interfere with my sport (I am very active) and I am worried about my GCSEs. It takes ages to get going in the mornings.

Assessment	Good	Adequate	Poor/not done
1 Appropriate introduction (full name and role)	☐	☐	☐
2 Explains purpose of interview	☐	☐	☐
3 Establishes nature and duration of presenting complaint	☐	☐	☐
4 Establishes the characteristics of the back pain: *Site – cervical, thoracic, lumbar, sacroiliac*	☐	☐	☐
Radiation – excludes radiation down the lower limbs	☐	☐	☐
Exacerbating and relieving factors	☐	☐	☐
Early morning stiffness	☐	☐	☐
5 Establishes/excludes peripheral joint involvement	☐	☐	☐

6 Establishes/excludes associated systemic symptoms:

Diarrhoea and GI symptoms ☐ ☐ ☐

Eye/visual problems ☐ ☐ ☐

Respiratory symptoms ☐ ☐ ☐

Urogenital symptoms ☐ ☐ ☐

General systemic symptoms ☐ ☐ ☐

7 Establishes family history – particularly of arthritis, IBD and psoriasis ☐ ☐ ☐

8 Establishes previous medical history ☐ ☐ ☐

9 Elicits patient's concerns and responds sensitively ☐ ☐ ☐

10 Appropriate questioning technique ☐ ☐ ☐

11 Avoids or explains jargon ☐ ☐ ☐

12 Summarises history back to patient, including concerns ☐ ☐ ☐

13 Makes a reasonable attempt at the diagnosis ☐ ☐ ☐

14 Systematic, organised approach ☐ ☐ ☐

SP to Mark

15 This student was understanding ☐ ☐ ☐

Diagnosis
Ankylosing spondylitis

STATION 3.3

Patient history

I am 27 years old and work as a supermarket manager. I am usually fit and well but I have developed a red, raised rash over both my cheeks over the past 4–5 months. The rash is slowly enlarging across the cheeks but has not spread to any other sites. The rash is not itchy or painful. I did have a nasty sunburn at the start of the summer but this has not recurred, mainly as I have avoided the sunlight. I have had painful joints in both my hands and feet but have not had any acute swelling or other signs of acute arthritis. No other joints are affected.

I have been feeling generally weak and tired, and have noticed over the last few weeks that my ankles, hands and face are swelling. I have also had a dull but persistent headache. I have been passing very little urine over the past week. I've had no eye, breathing or stomach problems.

I've had 3 or 4 DVTs in my legs over the past five years and am on long-term warfarin treatment. I have been married for four years and have had three miscarriages since. I am otherwise well and have had no admissions to hospital. Other than the warfarin I only take paracetamol for my headache. There are no family medical problems of note. I feel self-conscious about my face. I am awfully worried about what might be wrong. I am desperate to have a baby and am attending the recurrent miscarriage clinic.

Assessment	Good	Adequate	Poor/not done
1 Appropriate introduction (full name and role)	☐	☐	☐
2 Explains purpose of interview and gains consent	☐	☐	☐
3 Establishes reason for patient's visit	☐	☐	☐
4 Establishes duration and nature of symptoms	☐	☐	☐
5 Establishes characteristics of the rash: site, spread appearance, pruritus	☐	☐	☐
6 Establishes nature of the joint involvement:			
Excludes symptoms of acute arthritis	☐	☐	☐
Establishes joints involved	☐	☐	☐

Answers

7 Establishes/excludes:

   Systemic symptoms □ □ □

   Eye/visual symptoms □ □ □

   Respiratory symptoms □ □ □

   Upper and lower GI symptoms □ □ □

   Urogenital symptoms □ □ □

   General symptoms: headache
   peripheral oedema, malaise □ □ □

8 Establishes family history □ □ □

9 Establishes previous medical history –
  particularly recurrent DVT and several
  miscarriages □ □ □

10 Establishes medication history □ □ □

11 Elicits patient's concerns and
   responds sensitively □ □ □

12 Appropriate questioning technique □ □ □

13 Avoids or explains jargon □ □ □

14 Summarises history back to patient,
   including concerns □ □ □

15 Makes a reasonable attempt at the
   diagnosis □ □ □

16 Systematic, organised approach □ □ □

SP to Mark

17 The student was empathic □ □ □

Diagnosis
Systemic lupus erythematosus with anticardiolipin antibody. Symptoms suggest nephrotic syndrome and hypertension

Comment
Various syndromes within the broader diagnosis of SLE have now been characterised by the presence of specific antibodies.

Syndrome	Antibody
Photosensitivity (subacute cutaneous lupus)	Anti-Ro/Anti La
Photosensitivity, nephritis and serositis, eg pleurisy or pericarditis	Anti-dsDNA
Neonatal lupus syndrome – splenomegaly, rashes, thrombocytopenia and complete heart block	Anti-Ro/Anti La
Arterial and venous thrombosis, recurrent miscarriage, thrombocytopaenia, central nervous syndromes – psychosis, cranial nerve palsies, headaches and atypical migraine	Antiphospholipid Lupus anitcoagulant
Drug induced lupus	Antihistone
Overlap syndrome – Raynaud's, myositis, cardiorespiratory features	Anti-RNP

STATION 3.4

Patient history

I am 37 years old woman and work part-time as a telephonist. I have been unwell for about eight months. Last winter I noticed that my fingers and, to a lesser extent, my toes began to get extremely painful and changed colour in the cold weather. They went pale, and then red and painful. Over the last two months my fingers have begun to swell and the skin has felt very tight.

During the last three months I have also noticed increasing problems with my swallowing. Initially this felt like a slight blockage to solids, such as bread and potatoes but has now progressed to liquids, and I am finding it increasingly difficult to eat and drink. I have had increasing shortness of breath on exertion and my exercise tolerance has reduced to 400–500 metres on the flat. I have no other respiratory symptoms.

I have no other stomach symptoms, gynaecological or urinary problems. I do not have pain in my joints or arthritic problems. I do have pain in my muscles and feel generally weak. I have not noticed any furrowing around the mouth or small spots around the face. I have recently developed a dull, generalised headache and some blurring of my vision, but have put this down to feeling tired. In my family history my mother had a similar problem with her fingers but is still alive and otherwise well. I am on no medications and do not drink or smoke. I am upset that it has taken three months to get the hospital appointment. I am worried about what might be wrong. I am surely far too young to be having these problems.

Answers

Assessment	Good	Adequate	Poor/not done
1 Appropriate introduction (full name and role)	☐	☐	☐
2 Explains purpose of interview and seeks consent	☐	☐	☐
3 Establishes duration and nature of symptoms	☐	☐	☐
4 Establishes characteristics of Raynaud's syndrome:			
Colour changes	☐	☐	☐
Pain on exposure to cold	☐	☐	☐
5 Establishes character and level of dysphagia to solids and liquids	☐	☐	☐
6 Establishes/excludes other features of systemic sclerosis and connective tissue disease:			
Swelling of fingers		☐	☐
Respiratory symptoms		☐	☐
Urogenital symptoms		☐	☐
Acute arthritis		☐	☐
Skin changes/rashes		☐	☐
Lower GI symptoms		☐	☐
Muscle pain and weakness		☐	☐
Hypertension – visual disturbance and headache		☐	☐
7 Establishes family history particularly rheumatological disease	☐	☐	☐
8 Establishes medication history	☐	☐	☐
9 Elicits patient's concerns and responds sensitively	☐	☐	☐
10 Appropriate questioning technique	☐	☐	☐
11 Avoids or explains jargon	☐	☐	☐

12 Summarises history back to patient,
    including concerns   ☐   ☐   ☐

13 Makes a reasonable attempt at the
    diagnosis   ☐   ☐   ☐

14 Systematic, organised approach ☐   ☐   ☐

SP to Mark

15 The student was empathic   ☐   ☐   ☐

Diagnosis
Diffuse cutaneous systemic sclerosis

Comment
The initial advice to all patients with either primary or secondary Raynaud's
phenomenon should be to avoid cold exposure where ever possible and, when it is
not, to advocate the prophylactic use of heated gloves and socks. The patients should
be advised to stop smoking and avoid beta blockers. Short, uncomplicated attacks
may be treated with fish and evening primrose oil. Longer, more frequent attacks
may require the use of various therapeutic agents including calcium channel blockers,
transdermal nitratres, ketanserin, a selective $5HT_2$ receptor antagonist and ACE
inhibitors.

Severe attacks, which often are associated with ulceration, gangerene and secondary
infection, require hospitalisation and prostacyclin infusion, surgical debridement and
even amputation. Occasionally digital or cervical sympathectomy are required.

Answers

STATION 3.5

Patient history

I am 25 years old and have just returned from a holiday in Spain. After a bout of food poisoning about a week ago, I developed a hot, swollen left knee, which I am now unable to put weight on. I have no other joint swelling, but my buttocks and lower back are very tender and painful. My eyes have also been painful, gritty and red, and the lids are stuck together when I wake up. I have not had any visual loss. I have also had pain on passing urine, but no discharge. I have pain in my heels and ulcers both in my mouth and on the end of my penis. I have not had any rashes or other systemic upset.

My mother has Crohn's disease but there is no other family illness of note. I have had one similar episode to this one about two years ago, when I had a sexually transmitted disease after sleeping with a girl at a party. In the last 18 months I have been monogamous, but I am worried that my girlfriend might think otherwise. I really do not feel at all well.

Assessment	Good	Adequate	Poor/not done
1 Appropriate introduction (full name and role)	☐	☐	☐
2 Explains purpose of interview	☐	☐	☐
3 Establishes duration of symptoms and precipitating illness, ie food poisoning	☐	☐	☐
4 Establishes pattern of joint involvement, excluding sacroiliitis	☐	☐	☐
5 Establishes nature of eye problems, confirming conjuctivitis	☐	☐	☐
6 Establishes/excludes other symptoms of Reiter's syndrome:			
Urethritis, dysuria and discharge	☐	☐	☐
Achilles tendonitis		☐	☐
Keratoderma blennorrhagicum		☐	☐
Circinate balanitis		☐	☐
Oral ulceration		☐	☐
Plantar fascitis		☐	☐
Fever/malaise		☐	☐

7 Establishes sexual history and recent sexual contacts ☐ ☐ ☐

8 Establishes/excludes previous similar episodes – defining the precipitating cause ☐ ☐ ☐

9 Establishes family history, particularly of HLA B27 disorders ☐ ☐ ☐

10 Elicits patient's concerns and responds sensitively ☐ ☐ ☐

11 Appropriate questioning technique ☐ ☐ ☐

12 Avoids or explains jargon ☐ ☐ ☐

13 Summarises history back to patient, including concerns ☐ ☐ ☐

14 Makes a reasonable attempt at a diagnosis ☐ ☐ ☐

15 Systematic, organised approach ☐ ☐ ☐

Diagnosis
Reiter's syndrome

Comment
Reiter's syndrome – is an HLA B27 related disorder, which is classically made up of the triad of athritis, urethritis and conjuctivitis. Other features include plantar fascitis, achilles tendonitis, keratoderma blennorrhagicum, circinate balanitis, oral ulceration, acute anterior uveitis and fever.

The common precipitating factors are gastrointestinal and urogenital infections, including *Salmonella* (not typhi or paratyphi), *Campylobacter*, *Shigella*, *Yersinia* and *Chlamydia*.

Answers

STATION 3.6

Patient history

I am 65 years old and have been unwell for about two months. Initially I developed a dull, constant headache which was principally over the temples but has become more generalised in recent weeks. The headache is poorly relieved with paracetamol but I have not noticed any particular exacerbating factor. When I have the headache I also get a very tender scalp, which I notice particularly when I am combing my hair. Over the last month I have also developed a painful, tender and stiff shoulder and upper thigh muscles. The stiffness is particularly bad in the mornings and I've had to roll out of bed in the last few weeks. Sometimes my husband has to help me. I have not noticed any weakness or wasting of my muscles.

I have been getting pain in my jaw and tongue when I talk and while chewing. I have not had any visual disturbances, angina, abdominal pain or cerebrovascular symptoms. Over the past month I have lost my appetite and have lost 5 kg in weight. I have had no other systemic symptoms. I am worried that this could be a brain tumour.

Assessment	Good	Adequate	Poor/not done
1 Appropriate introduction (full name and role)	☐	☐	☐
2 Establishes reason for patient's visit	☐	☐	☐
3 Establishes duration of the presenting complaint	☐	☐	☐
4 Characterises the headache:			
Site: bitemporal		☐	☐
Radiation		☐	☐
Chararacter: dull, constant		☐	☐
Exacerbating/relieving factors		☐	☐
Scalp tenderness		☐	☐
5 Establishes pain, tenderness and stiffness in the shoulders and thighs	☐	☐	☐
6 Excludes muscle weakness and wasting	☐	☐	☐
7 Establishes/excludes joint involvement	☐	☐	☐

Answers

8 Establishes/excludes symptoms
   of giant cell arteritis:
   Jaw claudication   ☐   ☐
   Angina   ☐   ☐
   Limb claudication   ☐   ☐
   Cerebrovascular symptoms   ☐   ☐
   Mesenteric/abdominal pains   ☐   ☐
   Visual loss   ☐   ☐
   Anorexia, weight loss, malaise   ☐   ☐

9 Elicits patient's concerns and responds
   sensitively   ☐   ☐   ☐

10 Appropriate questioning technique   ☐   ☐   ☐

11 Avoids or explains jargon   ☐   ☐   ☐

12 Summarises history back to patient,
   including concerns   ☐   ☐   ☐

13 Makes a reasonable attempt at the
   diagnosis   ☐   ☐   ☐

14 Systematic, organised approach   ☐   ☐   ☐

Answers

Diagnosis
Giant cell arteritis with features of polymyalgia rheumatica

Comment
The diagnosis of temporal arteritis should be confirmed by a temporal artery biopsy. However the risk of complications, particularly blindness, means that steroids should be started immediately. There is a 48 hour window between starting steroids and loss of pathological changes in a biopsy.

The recommended treatment is prednisolone 30–40 mg od until the ESR normalises, then gradual reduction depending on the ESR and symptoms.

STATION 3.7

Answers

Assessment	Good	Adequate	Poor/not done
1 Appropriate introduction (full name and role)	☐	☐	☐
2 Explains examination; gains verbal consent	☐	☐	☐
3 Places patient's hands on pillow; ensures comfort	☐	☐	☐
4 Candidate washes their hands using the alcohol handwash provided (no marks if candidate only expresses the need to wash if handwash is provided)	☐	☐	☐
5 Asks patient if they have any particularly painful joints or areas before starting – reassures patient	☐	☐	☐
6 Observes patient's hands – commenting on presence/absence of:			
acute arthritic changes	☐	☐	☐
pattern of joints affected	☐	☐	☐
chronic deformities including Boutonniere; swan-necking; Z thumb	☐	☐	☐
Other rheumatoid changes – dorsal guttering; ulnar deviation of fingers; MCP subluxation; wrist deformity	☐	☐	☐
nail changes – vasculitic changes; psoriatic changes	☐	☐	☐
7 Asks patient to cross forearms over chest – commenting on presence/absence of rheumatoid nodules and psoriatic plaques	☐	☐	☐
8 Assesses function of hands:			
Gross motor – power of grip and making fists	☐	☐	☐
Fine motor – doing up/undoing buttons	☐	☐	☐

9 Assesses median nerve function:
   Motor – thumb opposition and abduction ☐ ☐ ☐
   Sensory – light touch over thenar
   eminence and palm ☐ ☐ ☐

10 Assesses palms for palmar erythema;
    tendon release and carpal tunnel release
    scars ☐ ☐ ☐

11 Completes examination by suggesting
    examination of other major joints and
    systems ☐ ☐ ☐

12 Ensures patient is comfortable and
    thanks patient ☐ ☐ ☐

13 Presents findings in a fluent, logical
    manner ☐ ☐ ☐

Answers

STATION 3.8

Assessment	Good	Adequate	Poor/not done
1 Appropriate introduction (full name and role)	☐	☐	☐
2 Explains examination; gains verbal consent	☐	☐	☐
3 Candidate washes their hands using the alcohol handwash provided (no marks if candidate only expresses the need to wash if handwash is provided)	☐	☐	☐
4 Observes patient – commenting on presence/absence of signs of generalised acute arthritis/chronic arthritis/other clinical stigmata of arthritis	☐	☐	☐
5 Asks the three screening questions of GALS	☐	☐	☐
6 Examines the patient from behind – correctly assessing and commenting on:			
cervical spine – extension		☐	☐
cervical spine – lateral flexon		☐	☐
cervical spine – lateral rotation		☐	☐
curvatures of the spine		☐	☐
rotation in thoracic spine		☐	☐
flexion in lumbar spine		☐	☐
symmetry of pelvis; sacroiliac joints		☐	☐
popiteal fossa – cysts		☐	☐
Achilles' tendons		☐	☐
7 From the side – assesses and comments on the curvature of spine; deformities at hip/knee posture	☐	☐	☐

8 From the front – assesses and comments on:

eyes – signs of iritis/conjunctivitis ☐ ☐ ☐

TMJs – pain and reduced movement ☐ ☐ ☐

cervical spine – flexion ☐ ☐

shoulders – place hands on back of head ☐ ☐

elbow – pronation and supination ☐ ☐ ☐

wrist – dorsi- and palmar flexion ☐ ☐ ☐

hands – grip power/make a pair of fists ☐ ☐ ☐

9 With the patient supine assesses and comments on:

hip flexion and extension ☐ ☐ ☐

knee flexion and extension ☐ ☐ ☐

ankle plantar and dorsiflexion ☐ ☐ ☐

Plantar surface of feet ☐ ☐ ☐

10 Completes examination by assessing and commenting on patient's gait ☐ ☐ ☐

11 Ensures patient comfort and dignity throughout; thanks patient ☐ ☐ ☐

12 Presents findings in a fluent, professional manner ☐ ☐ ☐

13 Examiner now asks:

(a) what investigations would you arrange? ☐ ☐ ☐

• FBC, U&Es, CRP/ESR – non specific ☐ ☐ ☐

• Specific – autoantibodies, eg rheumatoid factor ☐ ☐ ☐

• Radiology – X-ray of hands and other affected areas ☐ ☐ ☐

(b) What immediate management would you initiate? ☐ ☐ ☐

• Simple analgesia – paracetamol or NSAIDS.

Answers

STATION 3.9

1 True 2 False 3 True 4 False 5 False
This patient has a macrocytic anaemia and thrombocytopenia. The white cell count is normal but a differential should always be sought. The macrocytosis is associated with a reticulocytosis and hyperbilirubinaema which indicates haemolysis. SLE is associated with an autoimmune haemolytic anaemia. The thrombocytopenia is usually due to autoimmune destruction as well.

6 False 7 True 8 True 9 True 10 False
The data suggest this patient has acute on chronic renal failure. The hyperkalaemia is an acute marker whereas the metabolic acidosis, shown by the low bicarbonate, indicates chronic renal failure. The disproportionately raised creatinine to urea indicates renal rather than pre-renal impairment. SLE is associated with several different types of glomerulonephritis including rapidly progressive. The nephrotic syndrome is the triad of hypoalbuminaemia, significant proteinuria and oedema.

11 True 12 False 13 True 14 True 15 False
The data suggest the patient has a hepatitic jaundice which may be due to drug therapy or an autoimunne phenomenon. Gall stones classically cause an obstructive jaundice. The patient should have an ultrasound scan of the liver, biliary tree and renal tract in the first instance and then depending on the results a liver and renal biopsy.

STATION 3.10

1	(D)	(f)
2	(E)	(c)
3	(F)	(b)
4	(A)	(d)
5	(C)	(a)
6	(B)	(e)

STATION 3.11

1   (D) (e)

2   (E) (b)

3   (A) (c)

4   (B) (a)

5   (C) (d)

STATION 3.12

1 (D) (c)
Meningococcal bacteraemia usually causes a reactive, aseptic arthritis but may rarely cause a septic arthritis with evidence of bacteria within the joint.

2 (E) (a)
The aspiration from a gouty joint is normally aseptic with negatively bifringent crystals under polarised light microscopy.

3 (B) (e)
Pyrophosphate arthropathy or 'pseudogout' also gives an aseptic joint aspiration with positively bifringent crystals under polarised light microscopy. Radiographs may show intra-articular calcification.

4 (A) (b)
Spontaneous haemarthrosis is a relatively common complication of haemophilia, and prior to factor VIII transfusion caused severe deformity, sepsis and even death. Whether a haemarthrosis is spontaneous or traumatic one should never aspirate the joint unless under strict aseptic technique, some would advocate only in the operating theatre. Introducing sepsis into a bloodied joint provides a perfect culture medium for a severe septic arthritis.

5 (C) (d)
Reiter's syndrome causes an aseptic arthritis with a neutrophilia. The disorder principally affects the weight bearing joints of the lower limb, particularly the knee. It is usually asymmetrical.

STATION 3.13

1(a) True   **(b) False**   **(c) False**   **(d) False**   **(e) True**

This is a radiograph of rheumatoid hands. There is a symmetrical erosive arthropathy principally affecting the MCP and PIP joints. The MCP joints are mostly subluxed and there is evidence of periarticular erosion and osteopenia. There is also gross erosion and destruction of the carpus.

2(a) False   **(b) True**   **(c) False**   **(d) False**   **(e) True**

This radiograph shows gross changes of tophaceous gout. The arthropathy is asymmetrical and has caused destruction of the terminal phalanx of the right hand, with destruction and cystic changes at several of the DIP joints. The proximal interphalangeal joints are relatively spared.

3(a) True   **(b) True**   **(c) True**   **(d) False**   **(e) False**

This radiograph shows changes consistent with osteoarthritis. There is periarticular sclerosis and loss of joint space at the right middle MCP joint and ring and middle DIP joints. There are also changes at both first carpometocarpal joints. The PIP joints are spared. Arthritis mutilans is a gross destructive arthropathy seen in psoriatic and rheumatoid disease.

STATION 3.14

1(a) False   **(b) True**   **(c) True**   **(d) False**   **(e) False**

This radiograph shows gross degenerative changes of the right knee joint consistent with osteoarthritis. There is loss of joint space, periarticular sclerosis and osteophytes at the margins of the joint. The patellofemoral joint is almost totally fused (ankylosed).

2(a) True   **(b) True**   **(c) False**   **(d) False**   **(e) True**

This radiograph of a left knee shows intra-articular calcification. The principal cause of this appearance is pyrophosphate arthropathy which is a crystal deposition disorder, presenting in a similar manner to gout. The two are differentiated by their crystals. Pyrophosphate crystals are positively birefringent under polarised light, whereas urate crystals are negatively birefringent.

Other causes of intra-articular calcification include trauma and hyperparathyroidism.

3(a) False   **(b) True**   **(c) False**   **(d) False**   **(e) True**

This radiograph of a right hip joint and hemipelvis shows cortical thickening and trabeculation consistent with Paget's disease of the bone. There is no evidence of fracture. The patient would be expected to have a normal serum calcium and phosphate, with a raised alkaline phosphatase. Hypercalcaemia may arise due to fracture or concomitant malignancy. Cranial nerve palsies due to skull changes may occur and this may lead to deafness.

STATION 3.15

1(a) True   (b) True   (c) True   (d) True   (e) False
This is a lateral radiograph of the cervical spine clearly showing the 7th cervical and
1st thoracic vertebrae. There is loss of the disc space at C5/6 and C6/7. There are
small anterior osteophytes and evidence of degenerative changes in the lower
apophyseal joints. These changes are consistent with osteoarthritis.

2(a) False   (b) False   (c) True   (d) True   (e) True
This radiograph of the cervical spine shows atlanto-axial subluxation. The patient has
rheumatoid arthritis and this is a well recognised complication. The patient requires
neurosurgical stabilisation of the cervical vertebrae.

3(a) False   (b) True   (c) True   (d) False   (e) False
This AP film of the lumber spine and pelvis shows fusion (ankylosis) of the sacroiliac
joints and syndesmophytes causing the classical 'bamboo spine' of ankylosing
spondylitis. Such patients also suffer with ossification of the central spinous ligament,
leading to the tramline appearance. This disorder is associated with HLA B27.

STATION 3.16

1 (a) This investigation is a technetium 99, radioisotope bone scan.

(b) It shows multiple 'hot' spots throughout the thoracolumbar spine, ribs and
left scapula. This patient had metastatic breast cancer.

(c) The aim of treatment at this stage of disease is palliation. Bony pain may be
treated with local radiotherapy and/or appropriate analgesia. Other symptoms
arising from the malignancy and its metastatic effect should also be addressed.

2 (a) This is a plain (AP) radiograph of the pelvis, hip joints and proximal femurs

(b) It shows multiple lytic metastases in the pelvis and right femur. This patient
also had metastatic breast cancer.

(c) Lytic lesions are commonly associated with multiple myeloma and cancer of
the breast, bronchus, thyroid and kidney. Prostatic carcinoma produces both
osteolytic and sclerotic secondaries.

3 (a) This is a plain (AP) radiograph of the lower lumbar spine and pelvis.

(b) It shows a sclerotic wedged or collapsed fifth lumbar vertebra. There is also
loss of definition of the pedicle on the right, probably due to destruction. This
appearance is due to metastatic disease. There is a calcified mass lying to the
right of the vertebra which probably represents a calcified lymph node.

(c) Common causes of osteosclerotic lesions include localised Paget's disease of the bone, multiple myeloma and metastases from prostatic and colonic primaries.

STATION 3.17

1	(D)	(g)
2	(E)	(f)
3	(F)	(e)
4	(A)	(b)
5	(G)	(c)
6	(C)	(a)
7	(B)	(d)

Comment

In the treatment of rheumatic disease penicillamine and gold have a similar action and common side-effects such as skin reactions, mouth ulcers and blood dyscrasias.

Azathioprine and methotrexate are used to treat psoriatic arthropathy and are nephrotoxic and may produce lung complications.

Hydroxychloroquine and sulfasalazine produce liver and renal toxicity and hypersensitivity reactions including Stevens–Johnson syndrome (erythema multiforme). Hydroxychloroquine is avoided in pregnancy and lactation.

STATION 3.18

I am 36 years old and normally I am fit and well. However, I have not been well for the last week. Initially I developed a sore throat but this quickly spread to my chest and I am now coughing up thick yellow sputum and have a fever. Over the last 24–48 hours I have developed a severe rash all over my body. At first the rash was red and hot but has now started to blister. The rash started over my hands and feet and has now spread to cover much of my back and abdomen. I have also noticed there are blisters in my mouth, which has become very painful, and my eyes have felt gritty and sore. I have never had the rash before and have had no contact with a similar rash. I am on no medications, other than the contraceptive pill and have no drug allergies, although I am allergic to nickel.

I have no previous medical history of note and no other systemic upset. I feel in a panic about this as I have three children to look after and a part-time job. I've had to ask my mother to come and help. My GP got an immediate referral for me and I am anxious that something is badly wrong.

Assessment	Good	Adequate	Poor/not done
1 Appropriate introduction (full name and role)	☐	☐	☐
2 Explains purpose of interview	☐	☐	☐
3 Establishes reason for attendance	☐	☐	☐
4 Establishes duration and nature of symptoms	☐	☐	☐
5 Establishes the characteristics of the rash:			
Initial site of the rash		☐	☐
Sites of spread and effect	☐	☐	☐
Specific sites – mucous membranes and eyes	☐	☐	☐
Macular/papular/vesicular	☐	☐	☐
Associated erythema and heat	☐	☐	☐
Pruritus		☐	☐
Blistering		☐	☐

6 Establishes systemic upset –
   respiratory, gastrointestinal
   and urogenital   ☐   ☐   ☐

7 Establishes medications and allergies   ☐   ☐   ☐

8 Establishes previous episodes of similar
   rash   ☐   ☐   ☐

9 Establishes/eliminates recent contacts
   with similar rash   ☐   ☐   ☐

10 Establishes previous medical history –
   inflammatory bowel disease or
   rheumatological disease   ☐   ☐   ☐

11 Elicits patient's concerns and responds
   sensitively   ☐   ☐   ☐

12 Appropriate questioning technique   ☐   ☐   ☐

13 Avoids or explains jargon   ☐   ☐   ☐

14 Summarises history back to patient,
   including concerns   ☐   ☐   ☐

15 Makes a reasonable attempt at the
   diagnosis   ☐   ☐   ☐

16 Systematic, organised approach   ☐   ☐   ☐

SP to Mark

17 The student was empathic   ☐   ☐   ☐

Diagnosis

Erythema multiforme/Stevens-Johnson syndrome secondary to a chest infection

Answers

STATION 3.19

Patient history

I am 24 years old and work as a travel agent. I have been fit and well, although I am now very worried about a freckle on my left thigh. I first noticed it about 3 – 4 months ago when I seemed to catch it as I put on my jeans. The freckle seems to have got a lot bigger since then and has become more irregular and darker; the surface now feels quite rough. It is becoming increasingly itchy and because I scratch it, it has started to bleed. The freckle is now surrounded by other smaller but similar freckles but I have not noticed them anywhere else. (If asked: I do think that the glands in my groin seem quite swollen as well.)

Over the last year I have been taking part in body building competitions and as a result have spent 4–5 hours a week under a sunbed. I have always been a real sun worshipper and sunbathe when I can. I take at least three holidays a year, always to a sunny place and spend all the time I can on the beach. I have recently felt tired and run down but have been otherwise well. I am feeling terrified. I have read about skin cancer and know that freckles that bleed can be a sign.

Assessment	Good	Adequate	Poor/not done
1 Appropriate introduction (full name and role)	☐	☐	☐
2 Establishes reason for patient's visit	☐	☐	☐
3 Establishes when patient first noticed lesion/change in lesion	☐	☐	☐
4 Establishes specific characteristics of the lesion:			
Increased size		☐	☐
Change in margins/shape		☐	☐
Change in surface		☐	☐
Change in colour		☐	☐
Bleeding from lesion		☐	☐
Pruritus		☐	☐
Satellite lesions		☐	☐
Distant lesions		☐	☐
Local lymphadenopathy		☐	☐

Answers

5 Establishes the degree of previous and
   recent UV exposure ☐ ☐ ☐

6 Explains to patient concerns and reasons
   for referral to dermatologist ☐ ☐ ☐

7 Elicits patient's concerns and responds
   sensitively ☐ ☐ ☐

8 Appropriate questioning technique ☐ ☐ ☐

9 Avoids or explains jargon ☐ ☐ ☐

10 Summarises history back to patient,
    including concerns ☐ ☐ ☐

11 Gives clear, jargon-free explanation ☐ ☐ ☐

12 Avoids premature reassurance ☐ ☐ ☐

13 Invites questions, and answers
    appropriately ☐ ☐ ☐

14 Systematic, organised approach ☐ ☐ ☐

SP to Mark

15 This doctor was empathic ☐ ☐ ☐

Diagnosis

Malignant melanoma

Comment

Malignant change in a pre-existing mole is difficult to assess. However, a change in size, itchiness or bleeding, should arouse clinical suspicion. Delayed or missed diagnosis may result in dissemination.

STATION 3.20

A(a) False   **(b) True**   **(c) True**   **(d) True**   **(e) False**
This slide shows clubbing of the fingernails. There is loss of the nail angle and the nail bed is boggy or fluctuant. The nail demonstrates increased curvature in both transverse and longitudinal planes.

B(a) False   **(b) False**   **(c) True**   **(d) True**   **(e) True**
This patient has onycholysis which is a transverse splitting of the nail as it grows. The defect is associated with HLA B27 diseases and hypothyroidism.

C(a) False   **(b) True**   **(c) False**   **(d) False**   **(e) True**
This slide demonstrates onychogryphosis, which is an overgrowth of the nail. It is often associated with trauma, but may be caused by neglect, or rarely, ischaemia. It is a benign disorder.

D(a) True   **(b) False**   **(c) False**   **(d) True**   **(e) True**
The nails shown in this slide demonstrates the characteristic features of psoriatic changes. Abnormal growth leads to pitting and ridging and onycholysis. The patient may have plaques over the flexor surfaces but subcutaneous nodules are associated with rheumatoid arthritis.

Answers

STATION 3.21

Assessment	Good	Adequate	Poor/not done
1 Appropriate introduction (full name and role)	☐	☐	☐
2 Explains examination to patient and gains verbal consent	☐	☐	☐
3 Candidate washes their hands using the alcohol handwash provided (no marks if candidate only expresses the need to wash if handwash is provided)	☐	☐	☐
4 Correctly positions patient on the bed and appropriately exposes lower limbs	☐	☐	☐
5 Describes the lesion commenting on site, size, shape, surface, colour, condition of surrounding skin and presence/absence of satellite lesions	☐	☐	☐
6 Asks the patient if there is any tenderness; examines the lesion for tenderness, consistency, surrounding induration and mobility of skin over deeper structures	☐	☐	☐
7 Examines the remainder of both lower limbs for any other skin lesions	☐	☐	☐
8 Asks the examiner whether to look for other skin lesions over the body	☐	☐	☐
9 Examines both the groins for any associated lymphadenopathy; asks to examine for hepatomegaly and other lymphadenopathy – examiner stops them	☐	☐	☐
10 Repositions patient to ensure dignity. Covers and thanks them	☐	☐	☐
11 Provides a differential diagnosis of pigmented, benign and malignant lesions	☐	☐	☐

Answers

Chapter 4: Orthopaedics and Trauma Answers

Chapter 4:

Orthopaedics and Trauma Answers

STATION 4.1

Patient history
I have been suffering from a bad back for the past four years, and it is getting worse. It comes on when I lift patients or wheel heavy trolleys at work. The pain first started when I tried to stop a patient falling off a trolley and badly strained my back. It is now in the middle of my back and moves round to my hips. I am prevented from doing work in the house and was advised to lie on a firm mattress, which I do. I have had physiotherapy to my back, which helps only for a while. The pain is getting worse, and I think my back is permanently damaged and I should claim compensation. I do not think that I can do my job for much longer but I am not trained to do anything else.

Assessment	Good	Adequate	Poor/not done
1 Appropriate introduction (full name and role)	☐	☐	☐
2 Explains purpose of interview	☐	☐	☐
3 Enquires into presenting symptom (ie site, duration and radiation)	☐	☐	☐
4 Precipitating/aggravating/relieving factors	☐	☐	☐
5 Past treatment and results	☐	☐	☐
6 Asks about associated health factors; work-related stress; social/economic factors	☐	☐	☐
7 Elicits patient's concerns and responds sensitively	☐	☐	☐
8 Appropriate questioning technique	☐	☐	☐
9 Avoids or explains jargon	☐	☐	☐

10 Summarises history back to patient, including concerns	☐	☐	☐
11 Systematic, organised approach	☐	☐	☐
12 Makes a reasonable attempt at the diagnosis	☐	☐	☐

Diagnosis

Lumbar spondylosis

Comment

In patients over 40 years of age with long-standing back pain that is related to activity or posture, the most likely diagnoses are osteoarthritis and lumbar spondylosis. The latter is the result of disc degeneration (following recurrent prolapse) with displacement of the posterior facet joints. The unsupported movement in flexion and extension produces a form of segmental instability and may result in disabling symptoms. There may be neurological signs of an old disc prolapse (eg an absent knee or ankle jerk). Radiological features are characteristic of 'spondylosis'. Conservative measures, with management of pain, are sufficient for the majority of sufferers who are prepared to live with their problem. If, however, activity is severely restricted, surgical decompression should be considered. This may be combined with spinal fusion.

STATION 4.2

Patient history

I am a 38-year-old medical secretary and have been having attacks of severe pain and stiffness in my neck. I cannot think of anything specific that brings it on, except occasionally sudden movements or lying on one side. When I have the pain I am unable to hold my head up, and the pain moves to my neck muscles and goes down to my shoulder. The pain started about six months ago but I cannot remember hurting or straining my neck at the time. When the neck pain comes on I have recently felt tingling and pins and needles in my right hand, which slowly passes off after a few hours. My neck generally feels stiff and I cannot look behind me without the risk of bringing on the pain. It is affecting my work, as I have to lie down to relieve the symptoms. I am worried that I now have a chronic condition and it will not get much better. I want to start at a gym to get fit but don't see how I can do any exercise at all.

Answers

Assessment	Good	Adequate	Poor/not done
1 Appropriate introduction (full name and role)	☐	☐	☐
2 Explains purpose of interview	☐	☐	☐
3 Establishes presenting symptom site, duration and radiation	☐	☐	☐
4 Establishes precipitating/aggravating/ relieving factors	☐	☐	☐
5 Symptoms radiating to adjacent/ related sites (ie upper limb and back)	☐	☐	☐
6 Associated health factors: work-related stress, social/economic factors	☐	☐	☐
7 Elicits patient's concerns and responds sensitively	☐	☐	☐
8 Appropriate questioning technique	☐	☐	☐
9 Summarises history back to patient, including concerns	☐	☐	☐
10 Systematic, organised approach	☐	☐	☐
11 Makes a reasonable attempt at the diagnosis	☐	☐	☐

Diagnosis
Cervical spondylosis

Answers

STATION 4.3

Assessment	Good	Adequate	Poor/not done
1 Appropriate introduction (full name and role)	☐	☐	☐
2 Explains examination and obtains verbal consent	☐	☐	☐
3 Positions patient upright, facing forwards with arms by the sides and removes collar	☐	☐	☐
4 Asks patient to perform sequential voluntary neck movements and comments on discomfort/limitation	☐	☐	☐
5 Palpates spine from base of skull to T1 vertebra	☐	☐	☐
6 Whilst palpating asks patient to perform movements that are painful and comments on areas of tenderness/muscle spasm	☐	☐	☐
7 Palpates anterior triangles including trachea	☐	☐	☐
8 Completes examination, reapplies collar and thanks patient	☐	☐	☐
9 Presents findings in logical and sequential manner	☐	☐	☐
10 Attempts a clinical diagnosis	☐	☐	☐

Comment

The two common symptoms in the neck are pain and stiffness. Deformity usually appears as a wry neck; occasionally the neck is fixed in flexion. Numbness, tingling and weakness in the upper limb are due to nerve root or brachial plexus pressure, the former from a prolapsed intervertebral disc and the latter from a cervical rib. Cervical spondylosis (degeneration and flattening of the intervertebral disc) and disc prolapse (with nerve root compression) are the two common conditions affecting adults. Analgesia, heat treatment and rest (in a collar) are usually adequate for the majority. Traction in disc prolapse and physiotherapy in disc degeneration are effective in relieving more severe symptoms. Surgical fusion following evacuation of the disc space is seldom indicated in either condition.

Answers

STATION 4.4

Assessment	Good	Adequate	Poor/not done
1 Appropriate introduction (full name and role)	☐	☐	☐
2 Explains examination and gains verbal consent to proceed	☐	☐	☐
3 Correctly exposes both lower limbs whilst ensuring patient comfort	☐	☐	☐
4 Candidate washes their hands using the alcohol handwash provided (no marks if candidate only expresses the need to wash if handwash is provided)	☐	☐	☐
5 Stands at the end of the bed and comments on the presence or absence of deformity, swelling, normal skin but obvious muscle wasting.	☐	☐	☐
6 Palpation –			
• Asks patient for any tenderness, palpates round the joint margin for tenderness or swellings of ligaments and menisci	☐	☐	☐
• Palpates medial and lateral condyles of femur and tibia and surroundings of patella	☐	☐	☐
• Look for soft tissues, swelling of infra, pre-patellar or semi-membranosis bursae and Baker's cyst	☐	☐	☐
7 Examines for joint effusion by emptying the suprapatellar bursa and demonstrating the 'bulge sign' on the medial then lateral aspect of the knee joint. (If large effusion – by patellar tap)	☐	☐	☐

Answers

8   Movement –

- Ask the patient to actively move knee through limits of flexion and extension, comments on degree of movement and any limitation. ☐   ☐   ☐

- Examines passive movement carefully noting any pain examining limitations of extension, flexion and associated patello-femoral crepitus. ☐   ☐   ☐

- Examines rotation with the knee bent and looks for positive McMurray signs extending the knee from a rotated position medial or laterally. ☐   ☐   ☐

9   Examines for abnormal movement, laxity of medial or lateral ligaments – using appropriate technique ☐   ☐   ☐

10 Assesses the anterior and posterior cruciate ligaments by anterior and posterior draw signs (pushing and pulling on upper tibia when it is in the flexed position) ☐   ☐   ☐

11 Asks to walk patient to check stability and mobility and associated discomfort ☐   ☐   ☐

12 Measures muscle circumference, distance above and below tibial tubercle comparing the two sides ☐   ☐   ☐

13 Measures length on anterior superior iliac spine to top of patella and tibial tubercle and medial malleolus on each side ☐   ☐   ☐

14 Repositions patient to ensure dignity, cover and comfort and thanks them ☐   ☐   ☐

15 Presents findings in a fluent, logical manner ☐   ☐   ☐

16 Examiner asks – 'What do you think is the underlying diagnosis' ☐   ☐   ☐

Answer – osteoarthritis

Answers

STATION 4.5

Assessment	Good	Adequate	Poor/not done
1 Appropriate introduction (full name and role)	☐	☐	☐
2 Explains examination and obtains verbal consent	☐	☐	☐
3 Candidate washes their hands using the alcohol handwash provided (no marks if candidate only expresses the need to wash if handwash is provided)	☐	☐	☐
4 Observes patient's gait and stance and use of aids	☐	☐	☐
5 Performs Trendelenberg test and comments on joint stability	☐	☐	☐
6 Requests patient to undress to the underwear and lie supine	☐	☐	☐
7 Inspects for scars, sinuses and wasting	☐	☐	☐
8 Assesses skin temperature and palpates joint	☐	☐	☐
9 Measures limb length	☐	☐	☐
10 Tests for joint flexion (performs Thomas' test)	☐	☐	☐
11 Tests for abduction and adduction (prevents pelvic tilt)	☐	☐	☐
12 Tests for rotation with hips extended and flexed	☐	☐	☐
13 Tests for telescoping (abnormal movement)	☐	☐	☐
14 Requests patient to lie prone and inspects for scars, sinuses and wasting	☐	☐	☐
15 Palpates muscle bulk and tension	☐	☐	☐
16 Concludes examination by thanking patient	☐	☐	☐
17 Presents findings in orderly, logical manner	☐	☐	☐

Comment

When the patient walks into the consulting room, note the gait and any form of support used.

A limp may be due to pain, limb shortening or abductor weakness.

The Trendelenberg test assesses stability: the patient stands unassisted on each leg by bending the other knee. Bearing weight on an unstable hip results in the pelvis tilting to the unsupported side with the trunk compensating by tilting to the side bearing the weight.

The test is positive in:

(a) dislocation/subluxation of hip

(b) abductor weakness

(c) shortening of femoral head

(d) inflammation of the joint (osteoarthritis)

Limb length is the distance from the anterior superior iliac spine to the medial malleolus with both limbs extended. Shortening is identified either above or below the knee by flexing both knees with the heels together.

The Thomas' test unmasks a fixed in turn flexion deformity by preventing lumbar lordosis during hip flexion. This is done by flexing both hips to the maximum and then lowering one leg to the couch (normal range 130 degrees).

In abduction the pelvis is prevented from tilting sideways by placing the other hip in full abduction, checking that the pelvis is level. The hip being examined is now moved into abduction (normal range 40 degrees).

Adduction is tested by crossing one leg over the other, ensuring that the pelvis is kept level (normal range 30 degrees). Rotation is with the hip extended and the ankles rotated and noting the patellar excursions; the flexed hip is rotated by first flexing the hip and the knee to 90 degrees. Restricted internal rotation of the flexed hip suggests disease of the femoral head (avascular necrosis) or a torn acetabular labrum.

STATION 4.6

Assessment	Good	Adequate	Poor/not done
1 Appropriate introduction (full name and role)	☐	☐	☐
2 Explains examination and obtains verbal consent	☐	☐	☐
3 Candidate washes their hands using the alcohol handwash provided (no marks if candidate only expresses the need to wash if handwash is provided)	☐	☐	☐
4 Asks patient to uncover upper body, retaining underwear	☐	☐	☐
5 Inspects shoulders from front and behind for scars, sinuses, wasting and deformity	☐	☐	☐
6 Palpates shoulder to check for normal contours	☐	☐	☐
7 Requests patient to move arm and observes from front and then from behind	☐	☐	☐
8 Flexion and extension: asks patient to raise arms forwards and then backwards	☐	☐	☐
9 Abduction: asks patient to lift arm to the side and observes from the back. Tests for passive abduction by fixing the scapula and comments on glenohumeral movement	☐	☐	☐
10 Adduction: asks patient to move arm across the front on the body and rotates hand behind head and behind back	☐	☐	☐
11 Tests for shoulder power, asks patient to perform the following:			
• Deltoid – abduct against resistance	☐	☐	☐
• Serratus anterior – push against wall and check for scapular prominence	☐	☐	☐
• Pectoralis major – hands on hips and firmly push inwards	☐	☐	☐

| 12 Concludes examination and thanks patient | ☐ | ☐ | ☐ |
| 13 Presents findings in a logical sequence | ☐ | ☐ | ☐ |

Comment

Pain is the commonest presenting symptom in the shoulder and arises from any of the joints of the shoulder girdle or attached tendons. Referred pain may be from the neck, the heart, the breast or the diaphragm. When palpating it is best to start with the sternoclavicular joint and follow the clavicle laterally to the acromioclavicular joint and on to the anterior edge of the acromion and thence to the glenohumeral joint. Small changes in scapulothoracic and glenohumeral movements are best observed from behind. Abduction starts at the glenohumeral joint and when the arm is raised above the horizontal the movement is scapulothoracic which provides the last 60 degrees of abduction. This rhythmic transition of movement is altered by joint pathology and tendon dysfuction.

Rotator cuff syndrome: The rotator cuff is a sheet of tendons from muscles surrounding the shoulder that are closely applied to the top and sides of the shoulder capsule and inserted into the greater and lesser tuberosities of the humerus. Arching over the cuff is a fibro-osseous hood, the coracoacromial arch, with the subacromial bursa intervening. The rotator cuff syndrome is pain caused by tears of anterior and posterior muscles. Impingement of the supraspinaltus tendon with the arch is due to inflammation, tears, osteophyte formation and osteoarthritis of the acromioclavicular joint: abduction produces a painful arc, lateral rotation (palm upwards) allows the greater tuberosity clear of the arch and the remainder of abduction is pain free.

STATION 4.7

This is a Colles' fracture.

Assessment	Good	Adequate	Poor/not done
1 Technique for infiltration of local anaesthetic	☐	☐	☐
2 Technique of traction, disimpaction and reduction	☐	☐	☐
3 Maintenance of reduction and application of a plaster cast	☐	☐	☐
4 Post-reduction instructions to patient	☐	☐	☐

Comment

Although resuscitation and pain relief in multiple injuries take precedence over treatment of fractures/dislocations, there must be no undue delay in attending to the latter, as the swelling and inflammation that rapidly set in make reduction increasingly difficult.

Closed reduction: under appropriate anaesthetic and muscle relaxation, the fracture is reduced by a three-fold manoeuvre:

1 pull distal part in line with the shaft of bone

2 reposition distal part as the fragments disengage

3 adjust alignment in each plane. Alignment of the fragments is more important than exact apposition, except when the fracture involves an articular surface, when internal fixation may be required.

Answers

STATION 4.8

1   Glasgow Coma Scale

2   Pupillary size and reflexes

         Limb tone (and clonus)

         Limb reflexes

Comment

Unconsciousness following head trauma may indicate bilateral injury to the cerebral cortices, injury to the reticular activating system of the brain stem or increased intracranial pressure and decreased cerebral perfusion due to an expanding intracranial haematoma. Severe head injuries are usually admitted unconscious with a Glasgow Coma Scale score of 8 or less and require urgent assessment of the following:

A Airway – must be secured by a naso-laryngeal or oropharyngeal intubation. The cervical spine must be maintained in alignment until fractures have been excluded.

B Breathing – oxygen exchange is monitored and optimum ventilation with oxygenation is instituted to prevent hypoxic injury to the brain.

C Circulation – sources of extracranial bleeding are identified and controlled with volume replacement. Circulatory status is monitored by pulse, BP and CVP measurements.

D Neurological disability – presence of pupillary reflex, alteration in resting muscle tone, presence of abdominal, cremasteric and limb reflexes, Babinski response.

STATION 4.9

1	Patient	A	RTS	6
	Patient	B	RTS	10
	Patient	C	RTS	12
	Patient	D	RTS	8

2   Treatment priority in the following order: patient A, patient D, patient B, patient C.

Comment

Patients A and D are in severe respiratory distress and are both hypovolaemic. They require airway maintenance with cervical spine, ventilatory and circulatory support. Patient A, in addition, requires urgent head injury assessment. Patient B is moderately breathless and may have sustained a head injury. She requires a clear airway and oxygenated inspired air via a reservoir face mask. She requires further assessment for a head injury. Patient C is physiologically stable but not necessarily physiologically normal. An occult chest or abdominal injury, or even a head injury, may be present and she must, therefore, be observed overnight.

Answers

STATION 4.10

1   Extensive bruising over the lower back, extending to the right flank and abdomen.

2   Severe blunt impact to the side of trunk.

3   Injury to right kidney

       IVU

       CT scan (contrast enhanced of both kidneys)

4   Thoraco-lumbar spine

     Pancreas

     Liver

     Adrenal glands

Comment

Severe trauma may result in capsular tears or fragmentation of the kidney, and little if any bleeding is present per urethrum. Instead, severe haemorrhage occurs into the retroperitoneal space. Hypovolaemic shock is imminent, and the circulatory volume must be replenished. Continuing haemorrhage may necessitate surgical repair or nephrectomy performed as an emergency. Injuries that do not disrupt the pelvi-calyceal system, and in the absence of significant extra-capsular bleeding, may be managed conservatively; kidney function must be closely monitored. The patient is transported from the scene of the accident in a supine position, strapped to a long spine board with head and neck support. Following the ABCs of primary assessment, the patient is log-rolled to her left side, which is co-ordinated by four members of the resuscitation team. The back is examined for bruising and tenderness or numbness and muscle spasm. Radiology of the dorsal spine follows if indicated. Immobilisation is maintained until spinal injury is ruled out. Fluid resuscitation must be initiated when early signs and symptoms of blood loss are apparent or suspected. CVP measurement guards against over-transfusion.

STATION 4.11

Assessment	Good	Adequate	Poor/not done
1 Sandbags and tape; collar	☐	☐	☐
2 Application of a semi-rigid collar in neutral position sandbag supports to head and taped support to chin	☐	☐	☐
3 Inspection of neck for swellings, bruising and wounds: *Gentle palpation for tenderness*	☐	☐	☐
Spinal cord integrity:			
Test for motor power on same side (corticospinal tract)	☐	☐	☐
Test for pain and temperature sensation on opposite side (spinothalamic tract)	☐	☐	☐
Test for position and vibration sense on same side (posterior column)	☐	☐	☐
Spinal vertebral integrity:			
Lateral and AP cervical spine radiographs	☐	☐	☐

Comment

Patients with spinal injuries are often erroneously regarded as a 'specialist problem' and any deterioration activates urgent transfer procedures to a specialist centre without actively correcting spinal hypoxia and hypoperfusion. During the primary survey the signs and symptoms of shock should not be assumed to be due to the spinal injury. Even when a spinal cord injury exists, adequate perfusion must be maintained with oxygen delivery to the lungs to limit secondary neurological damage. Bradycardia with hypotension is not found in hypovolaemic shock and may indicate a cervical spinal injury in an unconscious patient; care should be taken to prevent over-hydration and pulmonary oedema by CVP monitoring.

Answers

STATION 4.12

Assessment	Good	Adequate	Poor/not done
1 Objectives: to identify and commence immediate treatment of limb-threatening conditions			
Group and cross match for blood transfusion	☐	☐	☐
Set up IV infusion	☐	☐	☐
Administer systemic analgesia (narcotic)	☐	☐	☐
Immobilisation: application of traction splintage	☐	☐	☐
Confirm neurovascular limb viability	☐	☐	☐
post-reduction (ie skin sensation, colour, pulses)	☐	☐	☐

2 **False (but needs continued monitoring)**

3 **True**   a, c and d

  False   b

4 **True**   a, c, d, e and f

  False   b

Comment

Multiply injured patients do not do well if non-surgical management of fractures involves prolonged periods of traction and bed rest. Early surgical fixation of fractures reduces pain and blood loss, and the incidence of pulmonary embolism and sepsis. Early mobilisation improves pulmonary function, promotes faster union and reduces infection. Trauma patients with limb injuries often have other major injuries that may require transportation to specialist centres. Traction splints may not fit some ambulances or helicopters, and the logistics of urgently transporting these patients must be worked out in advance.

STATION 4.13

1   Tibia and fibula; plate and screws

2   Internal fixation of tibia and fibula

3   a, b, c and d but not e are appropriately treated with this technique

Comment
In internal fixation a fracture is held reduced with transfixing screws or tension wires, which pass through the bone above and below the fracture and are firmly fixed to a closely applied plate. Complications of internal fixation are due to poor technique, poor operating conditions or poor equipment. They are:

- Iatrogenic infection which may lead to chronic osteomyelitis.
- Non-union if the bony ends are fixed too far apart (eg in the forearm and leg when one bone is fractured and the other remains intact).
- Implant failure, resulting in metal fracture when stressed across the fracture line.
- Re-fracture of the bone which may occur if the implant is removed too soon. Following removal the bone is weak and initially requires protection.

STATION 4.14

1   Tibia and fibula

         External fixator and tension wires

2   External fixation

3   **True** a, b, d and e

         False c

Comment
In external fixation a compound fracture is held reduced with transfixing screws or tension wires, which pass through the bone above and below the fracture and are firmly fixed to an external frame. This procedure is used for fractures associated with extensive soft tissue injury requiring the wound to be left open for regular toilet and/or debridement, inspection or skin grafting.

Most complications associated with internal fixation also occur in external fixation. More sophisticated external frames incorporate a system of hoops and tension wires to immobilise fractures, correct deformities, lengthen bones and transpose segments of bone.

STATION 4.15

1   Fig 4.15a: Fractured ribs and pneumothorax

2   Fig 4.15b: Disruption of the pelvic ring denoting a crush injury

        Fig 4.15c: Free gas in the upper abdomen indicating ruptured hollow viscus

3   **True** c, d, f, g

        False a, b, e, h

Comment

In the severely injured patient, treatment priorities must be established based on overall assessment. Immediate measures must consist of rapid primary evaluation, resuscitation of vital functions and then a more detailed secondary assessment and the initiation of definitive care.

The initial process is regarded as the A B C D and E of trauma care and identifies immediately life-threatening conditions as shown:

A   **A**irway maintenance with cervical spine control

B   **B**reathing and the need for assisted ventilation

C   **C**irculation with haemorrhage control

D   **D**isability indicating neurological deficit

E   **E**xposure requires completely undressing but preventing hypothermia

Answers

STATION 4.16

1   (a) Scoliosis of the dorsal spine

     (b) Primary lateral curvature – Cobb's angle

     (c) Idiopathic in the vast majority of teenagers
         Neuromuscular lesions in children
         Osteosclerosis of the spine in the elderly

     (d) Functional bracing with rigid pelvic and chin supports
         Surgical correction with rods and wires

2   **True**   a
     False b, c and d

Comment
The most common group is adolescent idiopathic scoliosis and it is usually found in girls. Lateral primary curves < 20 degrees either resolve or remain unchanged. Curves > 30 degrees are conspicuous and require correction or would otherwise progress. In this patient the lateral curve is about 30 degrees and requires functional bracing with a Milwaukee or Boston brace. Patients should be encouraged to wear it most of their waking and sleeping hours. Progress must be assessed four-monthly. Surgical treatment is reserved for failure of conservative measures or for severe deformities.

STATION 4.17

1 (a) False   **(b) False**   **(c) False**   **(d) True**   **(e) True**
This CT head scan shows evidence of cerebral oedema. There is loss of sulci and the 'ground glass' appearance of oedema. The patient would benefit from an intravenous mannitol infusion which would reduce cerebral oedema.

2 (a) False   **(b) False**   **(c) True**   **(d) True**   **(e) True**
This CT head scan shows a large right sided extradural haemorrhage. The extradural haemorrhage is produced by rupture of a meningeal vessel, such as in a boxing injury. Classically, the patient has a period of lucidity prior to becoming increasingly drowsy. The treatment is a burr hole through the skull to reduce the pressure and evacuate the clot. As shown an extradural haemorrhage produces a convex interface with the cerebral hemisphere.

3 (a) False   **(b) False**   **(c) False**   **(d) False**   **(e) True**
This scan shows bilateral frontal, intracerebral blood. Surgical exploration and evacuation of the blood clot is indicated in this patient due to the extensive nature of the frontal lobe laceration and deterioration of cerebral function.

4 (a) False   **(b) True**   **(c) True**   **(d) False**   **(e) False**
This is a lateral skull X-ray showing a large fronto-parietal fracture. CT scan is a better modality for imaging bone, MRI is better for soft tissue. This injury is consistent with blunt rather than sharp trauma.

5 (a) False   **(b) True**   **(c) True**   **(d) True**   **(e) False**
This scan shows midline shift towards the right with areas (white) of intracerebral blood. The patient should be treated with mannitol. Surgical intervention is not indicated immediately but may be required for obstructing hydrocephalus.

STATION 4.18

Assessment	Good	Adequate	Poor/not done
1 Skin preparation and draping Injection of local anaesthetic into surrounding tissue Wound cleaning, irrigation and debridement Skin suturing technique Wound dressing technique			
2 **True** b, c, e, h, i and j			
False a, d, f and g			

Comment

Wound management is aimed at optimal healing with minimal scarring and maximal recovery of tensile strength of injured tissues, with restoration of function. Adequate wound debridement cannot be achieved without preliminary infiltration with a local anaesthetic agent. However, heavily contaminated wounds requiring extensive cleaning or debridement require a general anaesthetic and are managed by secondary closure a few days later.

STATION 4.19

Assessment	Good	Adequate	Poor/not done
1 Identification of site of chest drain (ie 5th interspace, mid-axillary line)	☐	☐	☐
Skin prep and draping	☐	☐	☐
Infiltration of local anaesthetic	☐	☐	☐
Skin incision, insertion of chest drain and securing it with a suture tie	☐	☐	☐
Connection to water seal drainage bottle	☐	☐	☐
Suture of chest wound and application of sterile dressing	☐	☐	☐
2 A Pneumothorax	☐	☐	☐
B Right main bronchus	☐	☐	☐
C Collapsed lung	☐	☐	☐

Answers

Comment

Placement of a chest drain is an emergency procedure when an injured lung is being progressively compressed by air and/or blood entering the pleural cavity. The presence of haemopneumothorax rarely requires the placement of both apical and basal drains, as a single, correctly sited drain is adequate to drain both the air and the blood. Bleeding from a chest drain that initially drains 1500 ml or exceeds 750 ml in two hours usually indicates a significant vascular injury and requires thoracotomy for control. A tension pneumothorax presenting as an acute emergency may be immediately relieved by introducing a wide bore cannula into the pleural cavity.

STATION 4.20

1	A	Local anaesthetic, syringe and needle
	B	Central venous catheter set
	C	Giving set attached to IV fluid bag
	D	CVP manometer with 3-way connector

Assessment	Good	Adequate	Poor/not done
2 (a) Supine positioning of manikin	☐	☐	☐
Introduction of needle 1 cm below mid-point of the clavicle and advanced towards the suprasternal notch, thereby cannulating the subclavian vein	☐	☐	☐
alternatively			
Head down positioning of manikin Introduction of needle close to the medial edge of the sternomastoid muscle and advance towards suprasternal notch thereby cannulating the internal jugular vein	☐	☐	☐

(b) Withdrawal of venous blood into the syringe, removal of the latter, introduction of guide wire through the needle into the vein and removal of the needle ☐ ☐ ☐

(c) Venous catheter introduction over the guide wire into the vein and removal of the wire ☐ ☐ ☐

(d) Aspirate to confirm catheter in the vein by withdrawal of venous blood into the syringe ☐ ☐ ☐

(e) Secure the catheter to the skin with an op-site dressing; chest radiograph to confirm correct positioning and to exclude lung complications ☐ ☐ ☐

Comment

Shock is defined as an abnormality of the circulation that results in inadequate delivery of oxygen to vital tissues. Haemorrhage is the most frequent cause of shock after injury. The earliest signs of shock are tachycardia and cutaneous vasoconstriction. Thus an injured patient who is cold and clammy and tachycardic is in shock unless proven otherwise. Aggressive fluid resuscitation must be initiated when early signs and symptoms of blood loss are apparent or suspected. CVP monitoring prevents over-transfusion. The return of normal blood pressure, pulse pressure and pulse rate indicate restoration of the circulatory volume and the return of a normal urine output (30 to 50 ml/hr in an adult) indicates restoration of normal organ perfusion.

Answers

STATION 4.21

1   **True** a and d

         False b and c

2   A Litre of warmed saline

         B 1% lignocaine with adrenaline

         C Peritoneal dialysis catheter

         D Scalpel

         E Suture material

3   The catheter is inserted into the midline, close to the umbilicus (point X in
         fig 4.21b)

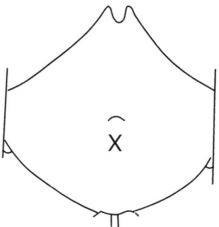

fig 4.21b

Comment

Diagnostic peritoneal lavage (DPL) is indicated for assessing abdominal visceral injury
when clinical examination is unreliable, for example in head injuries with altered level
of consciousness, injuries to the chest or pelvis, and with spinal cord injuries. Prior to
introducing a DPL catheter, the stomach and urinary bladder should be emptied by
nasogastric tube and urinary catheter to prevent injury to these structures. Following
instillation of a litre of warmed, normal saline, more than half the instilled volume
should be recovered in the ensuing hour. Failure to do so suggests a diaphragmatic or
bladder injury or, rarely, intravasation into a loop of bowel through a tear therein.

Mock Exam

The table contains five examinations of 19 stations taken from the text, each lasts two hours – this allows three five minute rest stations in examinations 2 – 4, and two in examination 5. The symbol + indicates a 10, rather than the usual 5, minute station, and ++ an extra 5 minute preparation for a 10 minute station. A 'subject' is needed to give the history, where this is provided in the text answer, and also for examination stations when stated.

Station	1	2	3	4	5
1	1.1	1.2	1.4	1.3++	1.5
2	1.10	1.7	1.8	1.9	1.6+
3	1.14	1.11	1.12.	1.13	1.16
4	1.19	1.17	1.18	1.15	1.20
5	1.21	1.22+	1.23	1.24	1.25
6	1.26	1.27	1.28	1.29	1.30
7	2.1	2.2	2.3	2.4	2.5
8	2.7+	2.8	2.9	2.6	2.15
9	2.11	2.12	2.13	2.10	2.16
10	2.17+	2.20	2.18+	2.14	2.19+
11	2.22	2.23	2.24	2.21	2.25
12	3.1+	3.2+	3.4+	3.5	3.6+
13	3.11	3.7	3.8+	3.9	3.10
14	3.16	3.12	3.14	3.15	3.13
15	3.20	3.18+	3.17	3.21	3.19+
16	4.1	4.3	4.2	4.6	4.4
17	4.11	4.5+	4.7	4.10	4.9
18	4.8	4.14	4.12	4.17	4.16
19	4.20	4.15	4,19	4.18+	4.21

The OSCE marking scheme

Traditionally, academic assessment has been 'norm' referenced, whereby candidates are compared to one another and are ranked from the best to the worst. In recent years the value of 'norm' referencing has come under question and 'criterion' referencing has become more accepted.

Criterion-referenced assessment is not new, the most obvious examples being the driving test and swimming life saving assessments. In both these examples a candidate must demonstrate a 'minimum competency level' for the given skills, ie driving a motor vehicle or saving a drowning person. Unlike traditional, norm-referenced assessment, there is no division of candidates into excellent, good, average, unsatisfactory and poor; there is only pass (competent) and fail (not competent).

Criterion referencing is easily applied to the OSCE format. A committee of examiners meets several months prior to the examinations and, through discussion, sets a minimum competency score, ie a passing score, for each given station. This score reflects what a candidate taking the OSCE should be reasonably expected to achieve, given their expected core knowledge, the time restrictions and the stress of the examination. These, in turn, should be reflected in the validity of the OSCE.

In volumes 1 and 2 the checklists are divided into three columns headed **Good**, **Adequate** and **Poor/not done**. These headings subdivide students into good, average and poor, where poor candidates do not demonstrate an acceptable level of competence, i.e. fail. However, in many medical establishments, the division of good and average candidates is regarded as old fashioned, regressing back to norm referencing and therefore the headings may read **Adequate or competent**, **Attempted but unsatisfactory** and **Not done**.

Some medical colleges apply weighting of individual items within a checklist. For instance, the initial item on each checklist 'Appropriate introduction (full name and role)', may have a maximum score of two marks if performed well, whereas another item, eg auscultating the four areas of the heart correctly, may carry 5 marks if performed well. Both would be given a lesser mark if performed adequately and 0 marks if not done at all. We have chosen not to weight individual items in our checklists. This is because:

(i)   We feel that weighting of items in this way does not improve the discriminatory power of the examination.

(ii)   We think students should be discerning enough to realise which are the important key points that will be more heavily weighted in a checklist.

We have, therefore, generally used 3 columns for our checklists, **Good**, **Adequate** and **Poor/not done**, carrying 3, 2 and 0 marks respectively. Certain checklists, however, only have 2 columns, i.e. Adequate and Not done. These are typically items which are required to be named, e.g. risk factors for a DVT or contraindications to a given treatment. One can only mention them or not and for this reason a 'good column' is not applicable. In such cases 1 mark is given for adequate column and zero for the Poor/not done column.

To obtain the total score

For each station, minimum competency or pass mark is calculated by a committee of examiners/experts. If a candidate scores each item as 'adequate' this will equate to the 'pass' mark. A candidate should therefore aim to get an adequate or good for each item. If one scores adequate or poor/not done in the majority of items, this implies a lack of knowledge or areas of weakness and should be used to direct the student's learning.

In most OSCEs the stations are deemed to be as important as one another, so that the mean pass mark of the total number of stations is taken as the pass mark for the overall examination. If individual stations are important in terms of 'must pass', a weighting system may be applied

to calculate the overall pass mark.

We have used one other style of marking whereby the station poses a series of questions to the student regarding an investigation, e.g. an abdominal radiograph, or a given scenario, e.g. management of a head injury patient. Examiners may consider that such answers should also carry serious consequences for the candidate, such as an outright failure on that question.

Establishing rapport with a patient is essential in a doctor-patient relationship. At the initial meeting, greetings and introductions help to put the patient at ease and ensure patient co-operation with the history and/or examination. In these stations, therefore, marks are allocated for such interaction. Positive criteria include empathy, putting a patient at their ease and establishing their confidence by careful listening and responding to verbal and non-verbal cues.

Revision Checklist

Cardiovascular diseases and Haematology

Arrhythmias ☐
Cardiac failure ☐
Valvular heart disease including endocarditis ☐
Ischaemic heart disease ☐
Pericarditis ☐
Hypertension ☐
Carotid artery disease ☐
Peripheral vascular disease ☐
Varicose veins ☐
Deep venous thrombosis ☐
Anaemia ☐
Bleeding disorders ☐
Thrombocytopenia ☐
Leukaemias ☐
Lymphomas ☐
Myeloma ☐

Respiratory Medicine

Asthma ☐
Bronchitis and emphysema (COPD) ☐
Pneumonias ☐
Pulmonary tuberculosis ☐
Bronchiectasis and cystic fibrosis ☐
Pulmonary embolism ☐
Pleural effusions ☐
Pulmonary fibrosis ☐
Respiratory failure and arterial blood gases ☐
Empyema thoracis ☐
Traumatic pneumo/haemothorax ☐
Bronchogenic carcinoma ☐
Diaphramatic hernia ☐

Rheumatology and dermatology

Osteoarthritis ☐

Rheumatoid arthritis ☐

Seronegative arthropathies ☐

Infective arthritis ☐

Lupus erythematosis ☐

Systemic sclerosis ☐

Systemic vasculitides ☐

Dermatological manifestations of systemic disease ☐

Nail and hair disorders ☐

Eczema ☐

Psoriasis ☐

Skin malignancies ☐

Orthopaedics and Trauma

Cerebral trauma ☐

Spinal injuries ☐

Thoracic injuries ☐

Abdominal trauma ☐

Pelvic and long bone fractures ☐

Bone dystrophies and dysplasias ☐

Bone tumours ☐

Spinal deformities ☐

Recommended Reading list

Medical Texts

Hutchinson's Clinical Methods: Hutchinson R and Swash M, 21st edition, W B Saunders 2001.

Davidson's Principles and Practice of Medicine: Edwards CRW, Bouchier IAD, Haslett C and Chilvers ER (editors), 19th edition, Churchill Livingstone 2002.

Clinical Medicine: Kumar P and Clark M (editors), 5th edition, Saunders 2002.

Lecture Notes on Dermatology: Graham-Brown RAC, Burns T, 8th edition, Blackwell Science 2002.

Examining Patients: An Introduction to Clinical Medicine: Toghill PJ (editor), 2nd edition, Edwards Arnold 1994.

Lecture Notes on Clinical Medicine: Rubenstein D, Bradley JR and Wayne D, 6th edition, Blackwell Science 2002.

Surgical Texts

Hamilton Bailey's Demonstrations of Physical Signs in Clinical Surgery: Lumley JSP, 18th edition, Butterworth Heinemann 1997.

Lecture Notes on General Surgery: Watson JE, Ellis H and Calne R, 10th edition, Blackwell Science 2002.

The Washington Manual of Surgery: Doherty GM (editor), 2nd edition, Lippincott, Williams and Wilkins 1999.

Bailey and Love's Short Practice of Surgery: Russell RCG, Williams NS, Bulstrode CJK (editors), 24th edition, Hodder Arnold 2004.

Obstetrics and Gynaecology Texts

ABC of Antenatal Care: Chamberlain G, Morgan M, 4th edition, BMJ 2002.

Lecture Notes in Obstetrics and Gynaecology: Hamilton-Fairley, D, 2nd edition, Blackwell Science 2004.

Index

Page numbers in normal text refer to the questions, page numbers in **bold** refer to the answers.

PASTEST – DEDICATED TO YOUR SUCCESS

PasTest has been publishing books for medical students and doctors for over 30 years. Our extensive experience means that we are always one step ahead when it comes to knowledge of current trends in undergraduate exams.

We use only the best authors, which enables us to tailor our books to meet your revision needs. We incorporate feedback from candidates to ensure that our books are continually improved.

This commitment to quality ensures that students who buy PasTest books achieve successful exam results.

Delivery to your door

With a busy lifestyle, nobody enjoys walking to the shops for something that may or may not be in stock. Let us take the hassle and deliver direct to your door. We will dispatch your book within
24 hours of receiving your order.

How to Order:

www.pastest.co.uk

To order books safely and securely online, shop at our website.

Telephone: +44 (0)1565 752000 Fax: +44 (0)1565 650264

For priority mail order and have your credit card to hand when you call.

Write to us at:

PasTest Ltd
Haig Road
Parkgate Industrial Estate
Knutsford
WA16 8DX